Syphilis and Subjectivity

Kari Nixon • Lorenzo Servitje
Editors

Syphilis and Subjectivity

From the Victorians to the Present

palgrave
macmillan

Editors
Kari Nixon
Department of English
Whitworth University
Spokane, WA, United States

Lorenzo Servitje
Department of English and Health, Medicine, and Society Program
Lehigh University
Bethlehem, PA, United States

ISBN 978-3-319-66366-1 ISBN 978-3-319-66367-8 (eBook)
https://doi.org/10.1007/978-3-319-66367-8

Library of Congress Control Number: 2017955042

Cover illustration: Samantha Johnson

Printed on acid-free paper

This Palgrave Macmillan imprint is published by Springer Nature
The registered company is Springer International Publishing AG
The registered company address is: Gewerbestrasse 11, 6330 Cham, Switzerland

Editors and Contributors

Editors

Kari Nixon is an assistant professor at Whitworth University. Her research focuses on the confluence of microbiology, germ theory, and social norms in the late nineteenth century. Her articles have appeared in *Disability Studies Quarterly, Configurations: A Journal of Literature and Science, Journal for Early Modern Cultural Studies,* and *Journal for Medical Humanities.* Her co-edited collection, *Endemic: Essays in Contagion Theory*, was published with Palgrave in 2016.

Lorenzo Servitje is Assistant Professor of Literature and Medicine at Lehigh University, working in the English Department and Health, Medicine, and Society Program. He researches the intersections of medical discourse and literature, focusing on the metaphorical militarization of medicine in the Victorian period. He also researches contemporary popular and technocultural representations of medicine. His articles have appeared in *Journal of Medical Humanities*, *Critical Survey*, *Science Fiction Studies*, *Literature and Medicine*, and *Games and Culture*. He has co-edited two collections, *The Walking Med: Zombies and the Medical Image* (Penn State, 2016) and *Endemic: Essays in Contagion Theory* (Palgrave, 2016).

Contributors

Shannon K. Carter is Associate Professor of Sociology at the University of Central Florida. Her research focuses on social inequalities, reproduction, and mothering. She is currently conducting research on African American mothers' breastfeeding experiences and peer breast milk sharing in Central Florida. Her collaborative research with Beatriz Reyes-Foster on peer milk sharing has been published in several outlets, including articles in *Breastfeeding Medicine* and *The Journal of Human Lactation.*

Nicole Cosentino is enrolled in the University at Albany's PhD program in English where she is studying queer theory and narratology in late 19th and early 20th century French, American, and British literature. She holds both a Bachelor's degree in Adolescent English Education and a Master's degree in English Literature from LIU Post. She teaches classes in composition, research, postcolonial literature, and queer theory; she also lectures on the works of Marcel Proust and Roland Barthes. She is in the process of writing her first book about queer literature of the 19th and early 20th centuries.

Monika Pietrzak-Franger is a guest professor in the English Department at Hamburg University, Germany. Her books include, as author, *The Male Body and Masculinity: Representations of Men in British Visual Culture of the 1990s* (2007) and, as (co-)editor, *Adaptations. Performing across Media and Genres* (2009), *Reflecting on Darwin* (2013), and *Women, Beauty, Fashion* (2013). She is preparing a monograph *Spectres of Syphilis: Medicine, Knowledge and the Spectacle of Victorian (In)Visibility*, which focuses on the visualization of the disease in late Victorian culture, for which she has received funding from the Volkswagen Foundation. In 2012, she was a visiting fellow in the Department of Anthropology at Washington University, St Louis. She has published on gender, medicine, visual culture and adaptation, and she is a co-editor of the journal *Adaptation* (OUP).

Beatriz M. Reyes-Foster is Associate Professor of Anthropology at the University of Central Florida. A medical anthropologist, she has conducted research on mental health in Mexico and peer milk sharing and vaginal birth after C-section (VBAC) in Central Florida. She and her collaborator, sociologist Shannon Carter, have published several articles on their work on peer milk sharing. Her articles have appeared in *Anthropological Quarterly*, *The Journal of Latin American and Caribbean Anthropology*, and *Critical Discourse Studies.*

Wendy Ryden is Associate Professor of English at LIU Post and Coordinator of the Writing Across the Curriculum Program. She has co-authored with Ian

Marshall *Reading, Writing, and the Rhetorics of Whiteness* (2012) and is co-editor and contributor with Monika Elbert of the forthcoming collection, *Haunting Realities: The Naturalist Gothic in American Realism* (University of Alabama). She is also co-Chair with Irene Papoulis of the national Assembly for the Expanded Perspectives on Learning (AEPL), an NCTE assembly.

JL Schatz is Director of Debate at Binghamton University where he serves as a lecturer and teaches courses on media & politics out of the English Department. He has published book chapters on the representations of apocalypse in the *Terminator* films, the construction of disability in the *Resident Evil* films, and the ecological security in the TV show *Lost*. Schatz has also published peer-reviewed journal articles on apocalypse and the environment as well as subjectivity in relation to teaching pedagogy in debate. He has also co-edited a special issue for the *Journal of Critical Animal Studies* and has been in charge of organizing several conferences, including the 13th and 14th Annual North America Institute for Critical Animal Studies and the 1st and 2nd Annual Eco-Ability Conference.

Joanne Townsend holds a PhD on Venereal Disease in Victorian Britain, from the Department of History, University of Melbourne, Australia, in 1999. Her essay, "'Unreliable Observations': Medical Practitioners and Venereal Disease Patient Narratives in Victorian Britain," has appeared in *Nineteenth-Century Gender Studies*, Issue 9.2 (Summer 2013).

Lisa Tyler is Professor of English at Sinclair Community College in Dayton, Ohio, where she has taught for more than 20 years. She is the editor of *Teaching Hemingway's A Farewell to Arms* (2008) and author of *Student Companion to Ernest Hemingway* (2001). She has presented at International Hemingway Society conferences in Stresa, Key West, Kansas City, Petoskey, and Venice, and has published articles on his writings in *Hemingway Review*, *Texas Studies in Literature and Language*, *Journal of Men, Masculinities, and Spirituality*, and half a dozen edited collections.

Livia Arndal Woods is a graduate teaching fellow at Queens College (CUNY) and a PhD candidate at the CUNY Graduate Center defending a dissertation titled "Heavy Expectations: Reading Pregnancy in the Victorian Novel" on October 30, 2016, under the direction of Professor Talia Schaffer. Her work has appeared in *Victorian Network* and *Nineteenth Century Contexts* and she will guest edit a forthcoming issue of *Nineteenth Century Gender Studies* in conjunction with the 2015 proceedings of the British Women Writers Conference, which she has co-chaired.

Contents

Introduction

Kari Nixon and Lorenzo Servitje

All diseases do cultural work. Syphilis has a particularly sordid history in this vein. Its specific etiology and symptomatology invited an array of (usually prejudicial) religious, political, and cultural uses. The disease took Europe by storm in the late 1490s, ever since then becoming a contested site of blame. Its venereal nature lent to its association early on with tainted sexuality. In the more medically advanced Victorian period, when a great deal more was understood about the disease from a scientific and public health perspective, it remained a prominent agent in shaping Western culture. As late as the 1880s, syphilis inspired hospital riots (Walkowitz 1980), punitive incarceration policies, and was surprisingly

K. Nixon (✉)
Department of English, Whitworth University,
Spokane, WA, United States

L. Servitje
Department of English and Health, Medicine, and Society Program,
Lehigh University, Bethlehem, PA, USA

K. Nixon, L. Servitje (eds.), *Syphilis and Subjectivity*,
https://doi.org/10.1007/978-3-319-66367-8_1

featured in a large proportion of artistic media, as novelists and playwrights featured it insistently in their work, leading one critic to complain that theaters had become "lazar house[s] with all…doors and windows open," portraying "on the stage matters that a blind beggar would hide under his patches" (qtd. in Matos 2008, 353). Many critics, Sontag (1979) most famously, have pointed out, all diseases have symbolic meanings and manifestations. For instance, while tuberculosis was often characterized in the early nineteenth century as an indication of a "romantic" or sensitive spirit, possibly triggered by heartbreak, typhus, on the other hand, famously contrasted against tuberculosis in *Jane Eyre* (1847), viewed as a disease of poverty and overcrowding, with clear class-markers attached to its mythos. Both remained signifiers of the individual ill body, however. Also deployed as a marker of class, character, and early in the nineteenth century, religious judgment, cholera was at the center of the debate between contagionist and miasma theorists, and was often seen as evidence of the need for sanitary intervention in lower-class neighborhoods. We name these few examples to demonstrate that while every disease comes complete with its concomitant cultural valences and mythologies, often, these were seen as needs for public sanitary reform, as reflections of the individual character, *or* as catastrophic acts of God, akin to other natural disasters. Syphilis, we suggest in this volume, stretched the bounds of the cultural work of disease into broader arenas dealing with individual and global subjecthood in an increasingly interconnected world.

Today, we understand syphilis's biological ontology as one of the several diseases that stem from pathogenic members of *Treponema*, a specific genus of a corkscrew-shaped family of bacteria known as spirochetes. It became easily treatable post-penicillin in the mid-twentieth century, and was overshadowed as the focus of attention by the advent of the Human Immunodeficiency Virus (HIV) and, more recently, the Human Papillomavirus (HPV) in the popular and news media. The disease is rarely fatal today (Catterall 2013). But, before this, it was the most dangerous and feared venereal disease for nearly the last five hundred years (Quétel 1992). What qualities made syphilis such a prominent social and cultural force historically? What are the disease's contemporary resonances? Its ability to masquerade as other illnesses, for instance, lent it a fluidity that heightened its symbolic potential. Additionally, its contagiousness, proclivity to disfigure and therefore to publicly "mark" its victims, its horrific manner of death via dementia—all of these factors rendered syphilis a disease that was particularly malleable, and capable of bolstering a wide range of social prejudices, anxieties, and power structures.

And yet, given its notorious history in the disciplining and punishing of sexuality and its close ties to the history of unethical biomedical research, among other social determinants and effects, syphilis still has much to tell us about modernity and the subsequent legacies that followed the disease in our recent past and contemporary moment. Because of the biological realities of syphilis's different symptomatology in its different stages, in addition to being an obvious marker of perceived physical impurity, it quickly became imbued with broader identities such as nationality, race, and gender, and was often rather predictably repurposed to bolster extant stigmas associated with these categories.

Syphilis and Subjectivity seeks to broaden interdisciplinary scholarship on cultures of medicine by investigating how syphilis in particular has had a role in shaping modern subjectivity. Two areas of focus dominate most scholarship surrounding the disease: its emergence in the early modern period—along with the related Columbian question—and the Tuskegee Study. The significance of syphilis from the late 1400s to the 1800s marks its rapid appearance in the years following Columbus's return from the voyage to the New World. Historical epidemiology has been fraught with debate about whether Columbus brought the disease back from overseas. The most recent forensic research that examines morphological and structural evidence in skeletal remains, however, suggests that it was widespread in Europe as early 1320 (Gaul et al. 2015). Whether it came from the Americas or mutated into a new, less virulent but significantly more contagious strain, in the sixteenth century, the "great pox" took a stranglehold on Europe. From this point forward, the disease prompted numerous medical writings, autobiographical counts, legislation, exclusionary measures, and accusatory writings (Quétel 1992). Within Europe, its origin became a question of ethnic and national blame. It was always somebody else's disease: "The French Disease," "The German Disease," "The Spanish/Castilian disease," or "The Jewish Disease" (Gilman 2010), among others.[1] The history remembered by medical practitioners and researchers today, however, is not one of national but racial difference, one that is not centuries but only decades behind us, if only temporally.

As numerous accounts have documented, syphilis's most recent legacy left a festering wound in American medical history. The US Public Health Service studied syphilis's effects in its full course—including the disfiguring and neurologically disabling, and potentially fatal tertiary stage—on African Americans from 1932 to 1972 under the pretext of gratis health care and guise of treating the nebulous condition of "Bad Blood." In cooperation with Tuskegee University, the study enrolled 600 African American men from Macon County, Alabama. Those who had contracted syphilis were *not* actively treated with the miraculous antibiotic penicillin, which had been deployed all over the world to rid people of the affliction by the 1950s. The infamous Tuskegee Study ushered in a new era of research ethics that remain in place today, outlining guidelines for the Institutional Review Board (IRB) review and approval of any research projects involving human subjects. Both Harriet A. Washington's (2006) *Medical Apartheid* and before it, James Jones's (1981) *Bad Blood* have documented these social injustices and the unethical auspices that produced decades of suffering for the sake of medical data—a history poignantly captured in their titles. Scholarship in this vein has not only focused on bioethics, critical race theory, and social justice but also on medical communication and education, such as the residual mistrust of researchers and practitioners that remains in the African American community (Roberts 2008; Gamble 1997), exacerbated by the still problematic instances of race-based medicine such as the BiDil controversy of the early 2000s, as work in science and technology (STS) and critical race studies has suggested (Kahn 2014; Pollock 2012; Roberts 2011).

And yet, given the early modern history, the Tuskegee Study, along with the development of penicillin and Salvarsan that has been extensively covered,[2] the authors in the chapters that follow consider these significant moments in syphilis's history, while focusing on other specific periods and cultural formations that reflect how the disease shaped collective and individual identity and experiences. In this capacity, the authors look toward a mix of cartography, medical writings, literature, historical periodicals, and contemporary popular discourses such as internet forums and electronic news media. Broadly, in this volume, we consider subjectivity in the capacity of the sets of power relations that structure human beings as subjects, both as agents of their own self-formation and as targets of economies of being and ethical regimes as characterized by theorists such as Foucault, Rabinow, and Rose. We consider syphilitic bodies as they have been subjected to the interrelated practices of reproductive futurity, statistical calculations, regulatory biopolitics, eugenicist discourses, and normalized models of gender, sexuality, and race.

Indeed, although syphilis is often most famous for its ancient, medieval, and renaissance legacies, as demonstrated by the volume of scholarly work done on these periods and others predating the nineteenth century,[3] the tincture which syphilis acquired in the post-germ theory age of the Victorian era had vast implications for the modern identity that persist today. While its role as a visible symbol of transgressive sexuality remained across time, the advent of the germ theory—ushered in the 1860s and bolstered by Pasteur's experimentation in the 1880s and onward—introduced an era of epidemiological certainty and faith in medical science seen never before. The 1880s in particular saw a deluge of scientists struggling to make a name for themselves by discovering the next microbial pathogen specific to a particular disease—what Paul de Kruif dubbed the "Microbe Hunting Era." In this latter half of the nineteenth century, the society was infused with a hopeful sense that what could now miraculously be identified as the cause of a disease must easily precede an ability to put an end to that disease. Causation, it seemed, must retrospectively imply not only a correlation, but also a means of eradicating such correlative relationships by means of a cure.

Syphilis was no exception. Even before its bacteriological agent was discovered in 1905, the zeitgeist of the era left public health workers with a keen sense that this disease could be eradicated through proper sanitary measures. Namely, as the disease was predominantly thought to be sexual in nature, nineteenth-century public health mandates zeroed in on sex workers, who then supplanted the lepers of the eighteenth century as social outcasts, as syphilis became "the dreaded symbol of social contagion" (Walkowitz 1980, 93). Yet, this movement took traction due more to military needs rather than discoveries of cutting edge science. Statistics after the Crimean War indicated a rise in syphilitic infections of British sailors while at port, and for a still imperializing nation, this perceived dissolution of the virility and vigor of the nation's symbolic representation of strength and power—its masculine troops—was a cause of great alarm. In an attempt to stem the tide of syphilis, Britain passed the infamous Contagious Diseases (CD) Acts (1864, 1866, 1869), a medicolegal mechanism Joanne Townsend discusses in her chapter. This legislation allowed law enforcement officers to detain and present suspects to a military physician who could then forcibly inspect the genitalia of any woman suspected of being a prostitute—this essentially put any woman alone after dark without a male chaperone at risk for such measures. If deemed syphilitic, the women targeted by the CD Acts could then be kept in "lock hospitals" for up to 6 months at a time or until such time as they "recovered" from a then-incurable disease (Walkowitz 1980). However, given the investment of middle-class politics in the lives of the poor, traction in the feminist movement, and the eventual extension of the CD Acts, medical control over women's bodies became a point of articulation and contest for gender relations.

As germ theory developed, the ineluctable realities of venereal disease epidemiology became more well-known and more difficult to obscure. Suddenly, morally scrupulous housewives and their children began to bear what were now recognized as obvious signs of syphilis. Moreover, regulation of prostitutes by means of the CD Acts had little effect on curbing the spread on the disease, according to statistics of the period (Baker 2012). Clearly, prostitutes alone were not to be blamed for this disease; if it was capable of infiltrating supposedly pure homes, then the men trafficking these sex workers were equally as culpable in its spread, if not more so, as their role incorporated innocent children. Furthermore, if soldiers subtended the health and strength of the nation, children quite palpably represented its future, such that syphilitic children came to be considered one of the foremost horrors of the era—vividly present in *fin-de-siècle* novels and plays, including *Ghosts* (1882), *The Heavenly Twins* (1893), and arguably even *Jude the Obscure* (1895). During germ theory's ascendancy as the dominant etiological theory, by the 1890s doctors began to recognize the dangers of men infecting their wives, and possibly their children through congenital transmission (Spongberg 1997). Eventually, after much protest and outrage—including a journal devoted entirely to the subject of repeal—the CD Acts were repealed in 1886, an effort led by feminists like Josephine Butler, marking a significant moment in which women were successful in "taking back control" (Sparks 2010) of their bodies from the patriarchal medical establishment.

While the repeal of the CD Acts certainly represented a huge victory in terms of social justice in Britain, the specter of syphilis continued to loom large over issues of race and nationality as the twentieth century dawned and progressed, particularly in militaristic contexts. Health campaign initiatives from World War I and World War II warned recruits about the dangers of sex while abroad, using a variety of persuasive imagery that often depicted women as intrinsically foreign and dangerous. During this time the metaphorical militarization of medicine, which had begun to emerge as a dominant conceptual paradigm during the nineteenth century, surged as a tool of wartime propaganda. Syphilis became a weapon of the enemy, if not the enemy itself, and was portrayed as such: a villain sapping the vitality of American troops as it did in other countries and other wars, such as the nineteenth-century Crimean War.[4]

Obviously, even up through the mid-twentieth century, syphilis was capable of threatening the core of national ideologies about its citizenry—and their material defenses in international spheres— in ways that exceeded the boundaries of the individual body and instead had much to suggest about the body politic and its place in an increasingly globalized world.[5]

Our volume gestures toward new scholarly approaches that investigate disease in interdisciplinary capacities. By interrogating the motivations that engender habits of belief, thought, and conduct regarding the disease and notions of the self, we seek to demystify the ideological constructs concerning syphilis. The chapters in this volume also consider the material conditions that influence the reception of the disease and the ways it has been conflated with the problems of modernity. Viewing syphilis from an array of perspectives, we aim to assess the ways syphilitic rhetoric affects the relationship, both conceptual and real, among mobility, proximity, and geopolitical borders.

As we seek to track broad cultural meanings of syphilis, the volume will not be organized chronologically; rather, *Syphilis and Subjectivity* follows a thematic and methodological organization. Because our initial aim with this volume involved taking up the well-known considerations of how syphilis reflected attitudes toward race and gender throughout history and expanding these considerations to other subjectivity-forming narratives, the first part, "Structuring Syphilis," addresses the ways that syphilis *itself* was defined and conceptualized by both the medical and lay communities. Monika Pietrzak-Franger's chapter opens this section with force, exploring the ways that epidemiological mapping was put to task in defining what would come to be seen as vulnerable populations with respect to this disease. Pietrzak-Franger deconstructs the seemingly post hoc nature of epidemiological mapping, revealing the socially constructed nature of epidemiological science itself. The second chapter, by J.L. Schatz, follows up on these conceptual strains by exploring the ways that already extant attitudes regarding sexual intercourse have in fact shaped the very way our culture insists on binarizing disease as "venereal" or otherwise. Schatz considers the way that our very notions of disease states issue from our pre-existing cultural biases and affect treatment protocols and public health recommendations in our contemporary moment. In the third chapter, Joanne Townsend builds on these notions of how power structures affect what came to be classified as epidemiological fact as she demonstrates how syphilis played a central role in fears about physical degeneration and the future of the British Empire in the late nineteenth and early twentieth centuries. Townsend examines how this anxiety shaped governmental initiatives and committees and medical writings, specifically with respect to the 1904 Inter-Departmental Committee on Physical Deterioration. She follows by illustrating how British feminists used syphilis as a vital part of their critiques of the institutions of marriage and motherhood, which as they made clear, were vital not only to women, but to the future of the entire British race. Anthropologist-sociologist team Beatriz M. Reyes-Foster and Shannon K. Carter follow Townsend's history of syphilis and motherhood with a focus on the contemporary phenomenon of human milk sharing and banking through the lens of nineteenth and twenty-first century concerns about syphilis and wet-nursing. In illustrating the Victorian roots of contemporary attitudes toward lactation, they draw from various sources such as ethnography, surveys, and media representation. Reyes-Foster and Carter identify echoes of earlier concerns with morality and milk in present-day conversations, noting a surprising contrast between alarmist media representations of peer milk sharing and the way in which milk-sharing mothers understand the practice's risks and realities. This first half of this volume delineates cultural anxieties, stigmas, and associations that primary literary texts investigated in the second selection developed from, responded to, and, in the case of chapters "Marriage, Motherhood and the Future of the Race: Syphilis in Late-Victorian and Edwardian Britain" and "Suspect Bodies, Suspect Milk: Milk Sharing, Wetnursing, and the Specter of Syphilis in the Twenty-First Century"'s investigation of syphilis in the twentieth and twenty-first centuries, help solidify.

The second part, "Novel Infections," elaborates on syphilis's discursive functions in the nineteenth to twenty-first century by looking at literary treatments of the disease as they shifted from the Victorian to the Modernist. Livia Arndal Woods's chapter opens part two, presenting a reading of Sarah Grand's *The Heavenly Twins* (1893) that diverges from the standard context of the CD Acts, which is usually applied to this text. Instead, Woods reads pregnancy in *The Heavenly Twins* as an indicator of changing norms in heterosexual marriage and thus broader notions of hegemonic morality in the middle class. Continuing with an examination of the disease's influence on British literature, in the chapter "Unspeakable Horror: Outing Syphilis in Joseph Conrad's *Heart of Darkness*," Nicole Cosentino and Wendy Ryden suggest that Joseph Conrad's *Heart of Darkness* (1902) yokes together medical fears and problematic sexual morality with a global violence infecting self-congratulatory European benevolence and charity. Conrad's tale, they suggest, is both implicitly and explicitly eroticized as well as steeped in gothic representation of the hidden and the revealed to manage an unsayable "horror." Consequently, *Heart of Darkness*'s language parallels pervasive late nineteenth-century syphilis discourse that likewise relies on obfuscation and silences, resonating with the symptomatology of syphilis and perceived syphilitics, such as Nietzsche and Columbus, who might have served as models for the notorious Kurtz. Looking toward the American literary work of syphilis, Lisa Tyler's chapter considers how Hemingway paradoxically seemed to often "look the other way" in the face of syphilis in his narratives, rather than casting judgment that he would have been quite familiar with through his physician-father. Tyler argues that Hemingway represents syphilis as one of the many universal taints defining the very condition of modernity.

Historians and cultural studies scholars of medicine have similarly demonstrated time and again that the medical in general is a productive site of investigation for so many ostensibly "non-medical" aspects of life. Medicine has much to reveal about historicizing and theorizing the social world, in particular about power relations by virtue of its material linkage of the individual to the whole, and about "the necessity and danger of human contact" (Wald 2008, 2). Pathologization is perhaps the mechanism for marking difference par excellence. Given this tendency, we look to a disease which has been associated with the most intimate of contacts to the most bellicose: from sex to war, manhood to militarized nationhood, from research hopeful at its best and militantly utilitarian at its worst, revealing at all turns the duality of human interaction and desire for progress and ascendancy.

Notes

1. The "Jewish" nominative for syphilis was of course not confined to the early modern period but remerged as a central point of the medicalized racial propaganda of the Nazi regime.
2. The first effective treatment against syphilis was the organoarsenical Arsphetamine ("Compound 606") developed by Paul Ehrlich in 1909. This was followed by the advent of sulfa drugs such as Protonsil (sulfonamidochrysoidine) in 1932, which were effective on a broader range of gram-positive bacteria. On the history of antibiotics such as penicillin, see Podolsky (2015) and Bud (2007). On prior chemotherapeutic agents, such as Salvarsan and sulfas, see Lesch (2007).
3. On modern syphilis, see most recently, Losse (2016), McGough (2010). See also Healy (2001), Arrizabalaga et al. (1997), and Merians (1997). For feminist readings of British and French histories of the disease in the eighteenth century, see Spongberg (1997). Broader histories include the work of Allen (2000) and Quétel (1992). In her recent *Syphilis in Victorian Literature and Culture* (2017), Monika Pietrzak-Franger broadens the scope of the discussion by addressing the unexplored tensions between the

visibility and invisibility of the disease and thus addresses a variety of cultural and media practices that accompanied the evocation of syphilis in the Victorian era.

4. We do not mean to suggest that antibiotic pharmacology was not also concerned with battlefield medicine and non-venereal disease acquired from combat and travel. Here, we are focusing on the hygienic and infectious disease aspects of military medicine.
5. In Western culture, as early as the English Civil War, the prophylactic was used as a preventative tool in military medicine to mitigate the devastating effects of venereal disease of soldiers. Fahd Khan et al. (2013)

References

Allen, Peter Lewis. 2000. *The Wages of Sin: Sex and Disease, Past and Present.* Chicago: University of Chicago Press.

Arrizabalaga, Jon, John Henderson, and Roger French. 1997. *The Great Pox: The French Disease in Renaissance Europe.* New Haven: Yale University Press.

Baker, Kimeya. 2012. The Contagious Diseases Acts and the Prostitute: How Disease and the Law Controlled the Female Body. *CL Journal of Law and Jurisprudence* 1 (1): 88–119.

Bud, Robert. 2007. *Penicillin: Triumph and Tragedy.* Oxford: Oxford University Press.

Catterall, R.D. 2013. Neurosyphilis. In *Contemporary Neurology*, 375–389. London: Butterworths.

Gaul, J.S., K. Grossschmidt, C. Gusenbauer, and F. Kanz. 2015. A Probable Case of Congenital Syphilis from Pre-Columbian Austria. *Anthropologischer Anzeiger* 72 (4): 451–472.

Gamble, V.N. 1997. Under the Shadow of Tuskegee: African Americans and Health Care. *American Journal of Public Health* 87 (11): 1773–1778.

Gilman, Sander L. 2010. *Diseases & Diagnoses: The Second Age of Biology.* New Brunswick: Transaction Publishers.

Healy, Margaret. 2001. *Fictions of Disease in Early Modern England: Bodies, Plagues and Politics.* Houndmills: Palgrave.

Jones, James Howard. [1981] 1993. *Bad Blood: The Tuskegee Syphilis Experiment.* New York: The Free Press.

Kahn, Jonathan. 2014. *Race in a Bottle: The Story of BiDil and Racialized Medicine in a Post-Genomic Age.* New York: Columbia University Press.

Khan, Fahd, Saheel Mukhtar, Ian K. Dickinson, and Seshardi Sriprasad. 2013. The Story of the Condom. *Indian Journal of Urology* 29 (1): 12–15.

Lesch, John E. 2007. *The First Miracle Drugs: How the Sulfa Drugs Transformed Medicine*. Oxford/New York: Oxford University Press.

Losse, Deborah N. 2016. *Syphilis: Medicine, Metaphor, and Religious Conflict in Early Modern France*. Columbus: Ohio State University Press.

Matos, Timothy Carlos. 2008. Choleric Fictions: Epidemiology, Medical Authority and an Enemy of the People. *Modern Drama* 51 (3): 353.

McGough, Laura. 2010. *Gender, Sexuality, and Syphilis in Early Modern Venice: The Disease that Came to Stay*. Basingstoke: Palgrave Macmillan.

Merians, Linda E. 1997. *The Secret Malady: Venereal Disease in Eighteenth Century Britain and France*. Lexington: University Press of Kentucky.

Podolsky, Scott H. 2015. *The Antibiotic Era: Reform, Resistance, and the Pursuit of a Rational Therapeutics*. Baltimore: Johns Hopkins.

Pollock, Anne. 2012. *Medicating Race: Heart Disease and Durable Preoccupations with Difference*. Durham: Duke University Press.

Quétel, Claude. 1992. *History of Syphilis*. Cambridge: Polity Press.

Roberts, Dorothy. 2011. *Fatal Invention: How Science, Politics, and Big Business Re-Create Race in the Twenty-First Century*. New York: The New Press.

———. 2008. Is Race-Based Medicine Good for Us?: African American Approaches to Race, Biomedicine, and Equality. *Journal of Law and Medical Ethics* 36 (3): 537–545.

Sparks, Tabitha. 2010. *The Doctor in the Victorian Novel: Family Practices*. Farnham: Ashgate.

Spongberg, Mary. 1997. *Feminizing Venereal Disease: The Body of the Prostitute in Nineteenth-Century Medical Discourse*. Washington Square, NY: New York University Press.

Sontag, Susan. 1979. *Illness as Metaphor*. New York: Vintage Books.

Wald, Priscilla. 2008. *Contagious: Cultures, Carriers, and the Outbreak Narrative*. Durham: Duke University Press.

Walkowitz, Judith R. 1980. *Prostitution and Victorian Society: Women, Class, and the State*. Cambridge: Cambridge University Press.

Washington, Harriet A. 2006. *Medical Apartheid: The Dark History of Medical Experimentation on Black Americans from Colonial Times to the Present*. New York: Anchor Books.

Part I

Structuring Syphilis

Medical Mappings of Syphilis in the Late Nineteenth Century

Monika Pietrzak-Franger

From the mid-nineteenth century onwards, civilization and syphilization were brought together in the European mind. In Charles Louis Philippe's *Bubu de Montparnasse* (1901), frustrated, syphilitic and desirous bodies become fused with the urban spaces of Paris. In an unremitting frenzy, they evolve into the stuff of the metropolis. When Bubu, the eponymous protagonist, leaves a bar after an orgy of absinthe, he sees the world as himself (Philippe 2006, 22): "The world was like a man, innocent and pox-ridden, drinking absinthe on the terrace of a café" (Philippe 2006, 43). This hallucinatory vision is a gasp of relief that Bubu feels after his panic and inflated fear are attenuated when he realizes that his condition is quite common. Until recently, investigating syphilis mappings has been part of more general projects concerned with the geographical dimensions of sexual politics. Recent scholarship has spotlighted the local specificity of regulatory directives, positioned them in relation to continental

M. Pietrzak-Franger (✉)
Universität Hamburg Institut für Anglistik und Amerikanistik,
Hamburg, Germany

K. Nixon, L. Servitje (eds.), *Syphilis and Subjectivity*,
https://doi.org/10.1007/978-3-319-66367-8_2

projects and inspected their geographical patterns along with tracing their historical development and their function in more general gender, class and racial conflicts, and with reference to British nationalist and imperialist ambitions. Certain places have gained particular significance in these inquiries: colonies as a cradle of contagion; cantonments, brothels, docklands and ports as local spaces of principal visibility; lock hospitals as junctions of broader geopolitical networks. In these studies, the flow of bodies, their spatial distribution and disciplinary targeting have gained particular importance. Within this scholarship, the significance of medical geographies of syphilis has seldom been addressed. Incorporating these materials redirects the discussion and points to the transformation in the preventive measures directed at the disease, which, as in Philippe's novel, seems to have infected the whole world.[1]

The assertion that "[t]he world was like a man, innocent and pox-ridden" also seems to have served as a motto to the late nineteenth-century medical books, which began to map out the dangers of the disease despite the apparent decrease in its severity and incidence.[2] From the mid-century onwards, medical publications were engaged in the geopolitics of syphilis. Following a heightened historicist impulse, they set out to determine the geographical origin of the disease while also outlining the dangerous spaces of its current spread. Medical men of all sorts began to trace synchronic and diachronic maps of the disease, both of which had an identification and comparison of syphilis sites at their core. The study of syphilis etymology highlighted historical geographies of blame, which were fundamental to the conceptual heritage of the disease.[3] It spotlighted the extent to which the relationships between mobility, proximity and geopolitical borders were central to the perception of syphilis. In historical debates, which pivoted around the question of the pre-Columbian origin of syphilis, the presumed site of its origination was juxtaposed with a number of localities where its prevalence had been recorded. The new discipline of forensic archaeology padded the search for the 'primeval' site of the disease. Texts and bones were the objects of its study: historical geography of syphilis was thus mapped out on the terrain where corporeality, textuality, temporality and space were conjoined. Synchronic mappings of syphilis, on the other hand, were based on the identification of the prime sites of its incidence in the nineteenth century. At the time when, apart from venereal syphilis, medical practitioners recognized the existence of non-venereal and endemic types of the disease, such attempts were a means of communicating the dangers of syphilis transmission as well as of voicing one's own political position regarding the modes of its prevention. With the advent of modernity, with new means of transportation, changing urban landscape and new forms of capitalized labour, the disease threatened to destabilize existing material and social orders.

Taking into consideration medical publications on venereal and non-venereal syphilis, I argue that the post-1850s insistence on an 'innocent' spread of the disease betrays larger fears fuelled by transformations brought about by modernity. In the context of new production and consumption modes, in which syphilis became divorced from the sexual act and extended over (intimate) relations, any sort of exchange became pathologized and served to outline the perils of modernity. Together with medical maps of syphilis, these debates articulated the necessity of replacing the grand-scale isolationist projects with nuanced exercises in civic responsibility as the chief means in syphilis control.

Medical Mapping Practices

The rhetoric of proximity was instrumental to syphilis prophylaxis. In his popular compendium *Syphilis of the Innocent* (1894), Duncan L. Bulkley, physician to the New York Skin and Cancer Hospital, divides syphilis into *syphilis parvorum* (venereal syphilis) resulting from illegitimate sexual relations and *syphilis insontium* (syphilis of the innocent), acquired either during legitimate sexual intercourse or as a result of non-venereal or hereditary transmission. This cultural-moralist differentiation is accompanied by the distinction between sporadic, epidemic and endemic types of the disease, where the latter refers to geographically specific variations of the disease such as yaws (Bulkley 1894, 17). Although there was no unanimity concerning these divisions, medical literature distinguished between the innocent and the venereal transmission of the disease, which, although tentative, produced various geographies of syphilis and activated differing scripts of sexuality (cf. Pietrzak-Franger 2017, 34). Despite a number of discrepancies, these geopolitical projects used mobility and social interaction as the basis for the preventive policies they supported.

Irrespective of their political persuasion and various explanatory models they activated, the authors outlining the distribution of endemic syphilis offered hierarchical maps of its distribution. Such visual and textual maps established a relationship among geographical dimensions, morality and the degree of cultural development. In his classic *The Geography of Disease* (1903), Frank Clemow, for instance, regards syphilis as prevalent in nations "whose moral views do not prevent promiscuous and uncontrolled sexual intercourse" and who are "ignorant of the infectivity" of venereal diseases (1903, 432). Racial and class distinctions are thus inscribed on the map of the world distribution of syphilis. In this context, Laura Engelstein's argument that, in its endemic form, "syphilis served Europeans as an exact index of cultural deprivation" (1986, 1038) should be further qualified to include racial differences. In these writings, race and class were combined with alleged patterns of knowledge distribution in such a way as to ensure a degree of imperial mobility and attenuate the fears of travelling in the tropics while warning against too close a socialization with the native races.

Historical and geographical patterns of mobility were likewise central to the studies in the distribution of venereal syphilis. In a strong intertextual gesture, such geographies were based on previous publications. In *Syphilis* (1895), Alfred Cooper divides the map of syphilis incidence into Europe, Asiatic Countries, Africa and America, the latter of which he discusses together. His inability to clearly qualify the occurrence of the disease and to underscore its geographical differences is striking. Although he professes to "show that great differences exist with regard to the frequency of its appearance and the intensity of its symptoms" (1895, 11), this diversity, with a few exceptions, disappears in his fuzzy qualifying clauses. Syphilis in Northern Russia, the Baltic states and in Finland is "severe" and prevalent (1895, 11–12). In central Europe, it is "more or less common" but depends greatly on "social conditions," "crowding" and the "number of military stations" (11). Cooper's geography is comparative and relational, as he produces, although only vague, hierarchies of prevalence and severity. "The complaint is less frequent in Belgium than in France, and in France less virulent than in England" (13). India and China are regarded as common spaces of syphilis transmission, with the latter hosting syphilis of "extreme severity" (13). In Japan, although "extremely common," the disease is only "mild" (13). Although prevalent in Africa, it is exempt from the "central portion of [the] Southern" part of the continent (14); "[V]ery common" in South America, it is "said to be more common" in Mexico than anywhere else (14–15). "More," "very," "extremely," "particularly," "mild," "severe" and "rare" are the qualifiers that should but do not give credence to Cooper's geography. With the exception of Iceland, where the disease "has been introduced over and over again [...] but has never made any progress and has never taken root" (11), Antilles, "the cradle of the disease," where it is "particularly rare" (15), and among Native American tribes with little contact with the European settlers (14), syphilis seems to be everywhere.

Dependent on specific climatic conditions, Cooper argues, syphilis seems to be less severe in "southern and temperate climates" (1895, 16), but race, population density, sanitary conditions and preventive measures are further factors that decide on its prevalence and gravity (15). Ethnicity is entwined with geographical factors as is visible in Cooper's assertion that syphilis "is said to be especially common among the Jews of Galicia" (1895, 12). With these criteria in mind, Cooper claims that despite earlier preventive measures such as the Contagious Diseases Acts, "England deservedly has the credit of preserving syphilis and pheasants better than any other country" (12). Although more detailed, Bulkley's historical geography of syphilis indicates roughly the same spaces of syphilis occurrence and severity and is as relativist as Cooper's, with such qualifiers as "considerable," "relatively" or "greatest" (1894, 6) as the only indicators of the gradation in the disease incidence. He also cites the estimation that "in the United Kingdom there were at least a million and a half persons infected with syphilis during each year" (1894, 7–8). In view of their relativist nature, these attempts at delineating a (historical and current) geography of syphilis are questionable as cartographic practices aiming to offer a legible map of the disease's incidence and severity. At the same time, however, they are a viable, although vague, means of underscoring its prevalence and indicating mobility as the chief factor behind its grand-scale distribution.

Clemow, like Bulkley, highlights the role of contact zones and mobility patterns to the spread of syphilis. He suggests that the relative absence of the disease among South and North American and South African tribes can be attributed to the "little or no intercourse with the rest of the world" (1903, 444). He also blames early settler communities for introducing the disease to the places in the world where it had been unknown. Importantly, in this retort, Clemow associates syphilis with the colonialist attempts of 'developed' cultures and with the dissemination of their 'unhealthy' habits. He thus underscores a direct relationship between the degree of civilization, morality and the prevalence of venereal syphilis (1903, 445).

Principally, while the sites of endemic syphilis were generally associated with a low degree of civilizational progress, its venereal type was regarded as a concomitant with modern, 'corrupt' mentalities. Where racial and ethnic differences were considered as crucial to the distribution and prevalence of endemic syphilis, class, race and mobility were seen as the major factors in the transmission of its non-venereal type. As Engelstein makes clear, "European physicians invoked the threat of non-venereal contagion to deter the educated from casual contact with the unhygienic poor and to emphasize the unintended ultimate consequences of original sexual delicts" (1986, 170). These assertions echoed pervasive modernist and imperialist fears of contagion while at the same time attenuating them by proposing prophylactic measures, based on a variety of tentative geographies of syphilis distribution, as a means of ordering or othering.

The Body of the World and the Power of the Hyperbole

Syphilis classification can be regarded as another technology of mapping, which aimed at a differentiation of its transmission modes, and which was intertwined with the issue of blame attribution. Bulkley provides probably the most nuanced and rich classification of syphilis transmission published at the time. Through his subdivision of sporadic types of syphilis into *syphilis economica* (acquired in industrial, social and domestic interactions), *brephotrophica* (referring to child care) and *technica* (acquired in medical context), further dangerous spaces of potential contagion are outlined and brought to the reader's attention (1895, 13–20). Their variety, clearly demarcated in the accompanying diagrams, also serves as an argument for the ubiquity of the disease. Lactation, circumcision and accouchement become as dangerous as vaccination, infection through care-giving or dentistry. While these sites of infection could be, to a greater or lesser extent, conceived as inherently dangerous, Bulkley's differentiation also helps him spotlight unexpected spaces of contagion. Almost every type of domestic, social and industrial exchange becomes pathologized.

In the industrial setting, buccal and digital are the most characteristic modes of syphilis transmission. They constitute latently perilous occupational hazards for glass-blowers, weavers, musicians, servants, cooks, shoemakers, cashiers, druggists, laundresses, old clothes dealers or artificial flower makers. Domestic and social exchanges are even more hazardous, as they span almost an entire sphere of possible interpersonal exchanges: eating and drinking, use of tobacco, contact with various articles, active and passive contact among the family members. While kissing, scratching or pinching can be avoided, there is a sense of doom and perilousness that surrounds the overabundance of articles which are potentially precarious: from spoons, knives and forks, torches, cups, glasses and jugs to towels, sponges and combs, handkerchiefs, pins, canes and opera glasses. In this overabundance of possible sources of contagion, everything and anything can be dangerous:

> With a poison so virulent, and capable of being transported and introduced in so many different ways, endowed with the possibility, as far as is known, of being preserved for an indefinite period, the only wonder is, that cases of the *non-venereal* communication of syphilis to innocent victims are not even more common than they are known to be. (Bulkley 1894, 21; emphasis in original)

Bulkley's panic-stricken rhetoric, amplified by riotous listings, tables and synopses, evokes an image of the world that has indeed turned into a pox-ridden monster where no exchange is free from potential hazards of infection. The invisible enemy lurks everywhere and can endanger even the most innocent of interhuman relations.

Not surprisingly, the geopolitics of syphilis, evinced through tables, lists and case narratives, was also literally mapped out on the human body. In Chap. IV (1894, 35–106), Bulkley offers a consideration of his private cases categorized with reference to the corporeal geography of syphilis symptoms. "Lip, tonsil, finger, breast, tongue, cheek, eyelid, chin, hand, nose, ear, temple, neck, forearm, and sacral region" thus become markers of an embodied geography of non-venereal syphilis (1894, 35). The disease is no longer only identified with the genitals, as was the case with its early conceptualizations; it has now spread over the whole body. Its visible manifestation, the primary sore, the chancre, "an indurated disc or button" (Hutchinson 1887, 4), bespeaks a double danger: as the disease can be transferred though the rupture in the skin, the chancre designates the spaces of the body's permeability. At the same time, it also signifies the hazards of proximity and contact.

In Bulkley's work, the syphilitic body, the corporeal topography of syphilis initial manifestations, is a truncated body of the mass, a sum total of the 2000 cases under his supervision. Although there is no clear gender specification, Bulkley notes a slight prevalence of extra-genital chancres among men, which undermines previous observations concerning their higher incidence among female patients[4]:

> It has been already remarked that extra-genital chancres occurred with greater relative frequency in venereal clinics among females; in the present instance the statistics are drawn from skin clinics and from private practice in diseases of the skin. It would seem, therefore, that practically both sexes are about equally liable to this mode of infection. (1894, 37)

Two efforts become transparent in this exposition. The first is Bulkley's direct attempt to modify the existing opinion as to the gender distribution among innocent sufferers. The second, more oblique but not less forceful, is a class-based argument: it may be true that hospital cases, usually drawn from the working classes and the underclass, show a higher prevalence of extra-genital infection with syphilis among women; yet, his experience with private patients, the affluent middle and upper classes, makes it clear that well-situated men fall victim to the disease as much, although not more, than women. Andrew Smith argues that the late

Victorian era saw a particularly strong association of dominant masculinities with "disease, degeneration and perversity" (2004, 1). He also sees the tendency of medical men to conceal the role of the middle-class client in the transmission of the disease as a political attempt to preserve traditional notions of male identity, which, rather than severing the link between masculinity and degeneration, paradoxically highlighted it (2004, 94). Smith's argument about doctors' attempts at deflecting guilt allocation away from middle-class men and relieving them from the burden of responsibility in syphilis transmission finds realization in Bulkley's work, where he delimits the degree to which middle-class men were victims of syphilis *insontium*.

Importantly, Bulkley's corporeal geography is instrumental to his panic-stricken rhetoric. The "location of extra-genital chancres" maps out syphilis *insontium* on the body of the whole, Eurocentric, world. Extracted from the existing medical literature, Table III (Fig. 1) combines corporeal topography of syphilis symptoms with the geographical identification of its incidence. Lips, tonsils, chin, nose, trunk, anus, neck, gums and ears become juxtaposed with parts of the world where these cases of extra-genital chancres were reported: France, Belgium and their Colonies; Russia, Poland and Asia; Italy; Great Britain, Ireland and their Colonies; the United States and so on: the world map is recapitulated along the spaces of syphilis incidence. As the countries are supposedly grouped on the basis of research clusters and professional alliances of the authors whose work Bulkley incorporates in his findings as well as on the grounds of their geographic proximity and their political alliance, the uneasy tensions are produced by the contrast of the novel, often surprising national constellations and their actual geographic and demographic constitution.

By synthesizing cases occurring over time, Bulkley universalizes his chart. It becomes a veritable geocorporeal phantasm of the world as a syphilis-ridden body, where the porousness of the skin symbolically stands for the disconcerting international constellations.[5] In fact, national alliances presented here evince the world that has gone wild "like a man, innocent and pox-ridden, drinking absinthe" (Philippe 2006, 22). Colonies are crammed into unnameable parts of their colonizing states; isolated Italy proudly competes with the United States and Austro-

SYPHILIS INSONTIUM

TABLE III.

Table of Localisation of Extra-Genital Chancres.

	Lips.	Breast and Nipple.	Buccal Cavity.	Fingers and Hand.	Eyelids and conjunctiva.	Tonsils.	Throat; deep oral and nasal.	Tongue.	Chin.	Cheek.	Trunk.	Nose.	Anus.	Peri-genital.	Leg and Thigh.	Forearm.	Neck.	Gums.	Forehead and Temple.	Ears.	Vaccination	Cupping and Phlebotomy.	Circum-cision.	Tattooing.	Total.
France, Belgium, and Colonies.	777	236	165	109	159	132	97	89	88	66	36	53	69	21	37	23	32	18	14	17	368	—	10	19	2635
Russia, Poland, and Asia	229	345	447	50	70	56	107	19	16	9	47	13	8	10	9	4	4	5	6	—	13	311	119	—	1897
United States.	107	28	17	75	30	26	10	11	6	19	1	7	1	1	2	5	1	9	3	3	887	—	6	42	1297
Italy.	161	350	59	17	13	23	4	6	17	19	6	3	4	4	9	3	5	2	4	3	209	—	—	—	921
Austro-Hungary.	233	18	19	110	18	22	9	11	12	7	6	6	1	2	3	11	1	—	5	2	121	180	32	—	829
Germany, Switzerland, and Holland.	169	107	7	35	26	11	22	2	5	12	1	7	4	36	6	4	1	2	2	2	54	254	5	—	774
Great Britain, Ireland, and Colonies.	90	38	9	59	46	15	8	13	2	11	2	5	—	3	5	8	3	6	3	—	204	—	7	21	558
Denmark, Norway, and Sweden.	39	23	11	5	1	22	5	5	—	—	1	1	—	—	2	—	—	—	—	—	7	—	—	—	122
Spain, Portugal, Mexico, Brazil, etc.	5	3	—	2	9	—	2	1	—	2	—	—	—	—	—	1	—	—	—	—	—	—	—	—	25
Total,	1810	1148	734	462	372	307	264	157	146	145	100	95	87	77	73	59	47	42	37	27	1863	745	179	82	9058

Fig. 1 Bulkey's localization of extragenital chancre, *Syphilis in the Innocent* (1894)

Hungary; partitioned Poland continues to exist as an independent entity jammed between Russia and Asia.[6] Devoid of gender distinctions (breasts as a distinct category disappear from this synthesis), the word becomes a disjointed gender-neutral body exhibiting symptoms of syphilis. Threatened by an invisible enemy, clandestinely marking domestic, international and colonial patterns of migration, the world is like an innocently suffering Leviathan whose body is threatened by corruption.

Although Bulkley's cartographic endeavours produce no actual maps but rather graphs and statistical tables, they partake in many of the strategies and practices characteristic of the nineteenth-century medical mapmakers. Like medical maps, this table is a rhetorical device, forming an argument that the world has been dislodged from its actual geographical space and appears to consist of a series of sore body parts. The fact that Bulkley decides not to outline syphilis on a real map is telling: by providing numbers rather than cartographic gradations, he adds urgency to the existing cases. By clustering the phantasmatic national and geographical spaces, he also creates his own topography of syphilis constructing at the same time a hierarchy of incidence (and innocence?) of the nations and their inhabitants. Maps, as Pamela K. Gilbert argues in *Mapping the Victorian Social Body* (2004), arose from the necessity of surveillance and governmentality. They evinced the "essential similarity" of subjects, bodies and spaces (2004, xiv), which is precisely what Bulkley is doing by organizing the figures along geographical and corporal axes. Yet his method of conveyance also significantly differs from the map rhetoric: as they delineate the spaces of disease occurrence, maps also point to the ideal that, as Gilbert argues, is always already implied in the outlined spaces that indicate the ideal of geography unmarked by the disease. This tension between imagined utopian spaces and tangible outlines of occurrence turn medical maps into narratives of potential sanitary progress, which symbolize, in the distance between what is shown and what is implied, the ambitions of their creators (Gilbert 2004, xv–xviii). In contrast, Bulkley's universalized table does not offer hope for a better world, devoid of the disease. Rather, in its synthesis, it creates a space of palimpsestous, historical recurrence of syphilis. His book is founded on the rhetorics of repetition, where riotous listings, graphs and synopses are combined in a hyperbolic argument as to the prevalence of syphilis. The sheer number of tables and their compactness creates a semblance of urgency further reinstated by explanatory notes. The final synopses, followed by an opulent bibliography on the subject, annul the utopia of the world free of syphilis. The continence of the world's body cannot be achieved. An instance of animate filth—swarming minuscule organisms—puts the body of the whole world at risk as they constantly infiltrate its borders. Such an approach pathologizes intimate social contact and calls for a rigorous policing of interhuman proximity and international exchange.

Pox-Ridden Urban Sites

In medical geographers' and practitioners' narratives, spaces of interhuman exchanges are obviously and symptomatically constituted as nodes of contagion and infection:

> Syphilis is everywhere seen to be a disease more especially belonging to communities, and flourishing most luxuriantly wherever there is a crowding or massing together of individuals. For the reason that thus the elements for its propagation become more concentrated, and opportunities for its communication more common: syphilis is, therefore, most abundantly met with in cities, and its frequency is commonly seen to diminish in a pretty direct ratio to the suburban or rural character of the people. (Bulkley 1894, 3–4)

Although Bulkley mentions exceptions to this rule, like others previously did, he considers the city to be the main site of syphilis infection.[7] No longer the exclusive peril of the unfaithful and sinners, *syphilis insontium* turns the whole modern world into a potential, although diversified, space of contagion. In medical books, the city, and especially the metropolis, becomes a dangerous space of modern liberal economy.

The relationship between syphilitic bodies, technology and urban spaces was explored in literary and medical publications across Europe. In *Bubu de Montparnasse*, they coexist in an incessant frenzy of velocity and exchangeability. Paris stands for their interlocking and for the resulting frustration. Pierre Hardy, a naive émigré from adjacent provinces, Berthe Méténier, a good-hearted florist *cum* prostitute, Bubu—Maurice Bélu—her husband by custom and pimp by conviction, all three syphilitic, are described in terms of the city. Paris is like a prostitute, prostitutes are like Paris: enclosed by the steamy embrace of a sordid room, Pierre "pour[s] himself into a dirty girl as into a public sink" (Philippe 2006, 10). Berthe is like her room, devoid of light "in her yellowish slimness" (33). Paris is like Bubu: drunk and vertiginous. But it is Pierre, in his naiveté and a procrastinating, abortive awakening of conscience, who embodies the tensions and uncertainties of modernity. Although with little literary skill and disarming frankness, Philippe paints a picture of Pierre's crisis: draughtsman for a railway company, he attempts to live a life in the phantasmatic utopian Paris, whose realities are woven of the everyday suffocating incandescence of the mob, the animal cries of the inmates of the Broca Hospital, only seldom heard in the tumult of the street life, and of his quiet work as a clerk.[8] Paris, like any metropolis, incorporates both the ideas of progress and danger; it obviously becomes a centre for the tensions and crises of modernity.

Scholars have written abundantly about these seemingly incompatible yet inseparable qualities of the modern metropolis. In the English context, Judith Walkowitz (1992) attends to the frequent pathologization of London's streets in the last decades of the century. Acquainted with the equation between the city and the streetwalker, "a central spectacle in a set of urban encounters and fantasies" (1992, 21), she lends her ear to other constructs of London's space subverted or reiterated by middle-class and working-class women. Aware of gender geographies and addressing the new urban technologies of mapping, Lynda Nead regards London in its double capacity as a dangerous or progressive modern Babylon, "whose splendour was its downfall," a symbol of "material wonder and tumultuous destruction" (2000, 3), at a time when it partook in "a highly concentrated discourse on the modern" (2000, 5). Richard Sennett (1994) points out the urban development of London's spaces as founded on the principle of body circulation and respiration simultaneously highlighting the growing superficiality of its ornate architecture which, appearing in all its lustre, hides enclaves of poverty. Erika Rappaport sees in it a space that exposes and promotes new mechanisms of production, mass consumption and communication, a space of increasingly rationalized and bureaucratized labour (2001, 25). Like Nead and Walkowitz before her, Rappaport addresses the gendering of the discourses around London along with referencing the ways in which it became a space for new forms of entrepreneurial projects among working-class women. Pamela Gilbert (2004) takes up Nead's contention about the city as a "focused instance of modernity" (2000, 5), exemplified in the principles of mapping and movement, in order to outline medical and industrial attempts at policing the boundaries of the social body. She investigates mid-nineteenth-century sanitary projects that suggested utopian goals in their dystopian mappings. All of them discuss urban spaces in their antithetical quality as sites of progress and degeneration.

Like in Philippe's novel, in medical narratives of the time, modern urban space is infested with pox. With the increase of reports on non-venereal syphilis, urban spaces, irrespective of their wealth, become sites swarming with the disease: the slums and the docs with its venereal variation, tourist hallmarks, restaurants and public amenities with the non-venereal genus. The medical press was replete with reports of innocent cases of syphilis in industrial and professional settings. There was no point in mapping out syphilis spaces because spaces of modernity were inherently pox-infested, literally and symbolically. Syphilis had become the padding of modernity. The ever nuanced and expanding sites of its germination, and the frantic attempts at their delimitation, testify to the underlying fear of changes brought about by modernity, above all, the transformation in the interhuman proxemics: the ever disappearing distance between people, classes, ethnicities and genders that necessitated a formation of protective barriers. By using a hyperbolic rhetoric of mapping, medical men made the world, and especially the most immediate spaces of social and industrial exchanges, into a perilous landscape of syphilis contagion.

The Dialectics of Glass and Civic Responsibility

The perils brought about by *syphilis insontium* were also addressed in popular literature. Interestingly, in *Bubu de Montparnasse*, these concerns become closely associated with the (im)materiality and symbolism of glass. Infected with venereal syphilis, Pierre imagines his return to his provincial home:

> Every night, I'll be in the good warmth of the provinces which penetrates into our hearts and hatches our thoughts like little chickens. This is my first year of syphilis. I will kiss everyone and drink in glasses. And they'll say to Juliette: "Along with you, greedy girl, have a drink out of your uncle's glass!" [...] I won't know what to say about my glass. (2006, 84)

The imaginary scene evinces the powerful emotions of longing and regret that Pierre associates with his return home. He realizes what threat he constitutes to his family. The simple action of glass-sharing, the symbol of closeness and intimacy, is now associated with an overtaxation of these relationships.

This tension references the double function of syphilis in the book: its role as an embodiment of dangers of modernity but also, paradoxically, as an entity which helps establish more intimate bonds among people. Jean-Louis Cabanès sees these contradictions when he argues that:

> La vérole est ferment de séparation [...] elle établit également des liens, une compassion. Si elle constitue un obstacle pour l'amour de Pierre et de Berthe, elle est non moins le catalyseur de leur union. [...] Faire l'apprentissage de la syphilis, ce sera donc accepter de la vie dans son ambivalence et dans sa plénitude. (1996, 105)[9]

The ambivalence of modernity, that Pierre encounters in Paris, the metropolis ridden with pox as it is ridden with great dreams of new developers, manifests itself in syphilis and in the glass that transports it. This contamination of modernity polices his actions and his intimate bonds. Schonlau argues that Philippe's novel cannot be regarded as an example of educational, social-hygienic fiction (2005, 342). While it is true that the novel in no way offers lessons characteristic of this genre, it is also clear that the lesson it conveys concerns the ubiquity of syphilis, with its central place in the modernist project. "We all have it" asserts Grand Jules astonished that Maurice might have just acquired it (2006, 39). Paradoxically, though, while it gives vitality to Maurice's milieu, the disease also envelops Pierre with a sense of inertia, of not being able to change anything. In general, Schonlau is right in claiming that the milieu-specific character of the disease, which, as part of the everyday toil of the underclasses, can hardly be regarded as acquired in a non-venereal way (2005, 343). And yet it also transpires that the disease is not constrained to specific classes or cityscapes, even as Philippe only highlights some of them. It can still be transmitted to other milieus.

Despite its strong anchoring in the French context and in spite of its considerable thematic and aesthetic individuality, the novel spotlights the growing preoccupation of the medical men with the ubiquity of syphilis.[10] The fears associated with the porousness of corporeal and social boundaries and with modern technologies were also an integral part of medical reports of syphilis transmission in industrial settings. In this context, glass, and glass-blowing, exemplified and symbolized these broader fears as well as highlighting the dangers of syphilis (in)visibility. Medical literature of the time abounds in examples in which either the process of glass-blowing or the joint use of glasses and cups are indicated as highly dangerous. Cooper's descriptions are typical:

> the secretions from the mouth of a person affected with syphilitic lesions of that part may adhere to drinking utensils, tobacco-pipes, and other articles used by several persons in common, and may thus convey the disease. Instances of this kind have occurred in glass factories, where one blowpipe is used by several workmen, and passed from mouth to mouth. (1895, 57)

Simeon Snell, the then president of the British Medical Association, recounts the story of a glass-blower who infected "more than four innocent persons":

> Seven years before consulting me he had worked as a glass-blower. He had to use the same tube as two other men. He developed what appears to have been a chancre at the back of the throat (tonsil). This was followed by a rash on the chest, and his hair fell off. At this time working with the patient was a man suspected by his mates of having syphilis the man in question denied that it was syphilis, asserting that it was *only* the "clap." The manager told my patient that he would take no harm, but he said, as a preventive he washed out his mouth with water. (1908, 1678; emphasis in original)

The infectious worker, who travelled to the neighbouring town, infected several men in the new factory, while Snell's patient communicated the disease to his wife. Generally, although Snell agrees that an indirect infection with syphilis is rare, he considers glass-blowing as a notable exception as its specific industrial context is favourable to the infection: the blowing pipe is passed from one man's mouth to another's without any precautions. Even though, according to Sommerfeld, syphilis amounted to no more than 1 per cent of all the diseases among glass-blowers (in Weyl 1908, 346), the sheer number of accounts printed at the turn of the century made it appear as particularly prevalent in this industrial environment.[11]

Demarcating glass-blowing as another, characteristically modern way of syphilis transmission had practical and symbolic consequences. Practically, it raised questions about the hygiene of the work environment, employment possibilities and rights to compensation for the infected. Snell, for instance, contended that "syphilis contracted in this way must be looked upon as an industrial accident, and would therefore be liable to compensation" (1908, 1678). Symbolically, this insistence on the dangers of the profession was much more complex and, like the relation to consumption, closely referenced the perils of modernity. Isobel Armstrong considers glass as the prime material of Victorian modernity, which induced ontological and epistemological changes in the world:

> Such a world, newly mediated by glass, was one of the projects of Victorian modernism, or, more exactly, a place where related and complex Victorian modernities played out their concerns. In the nineteenth century glass became a third or middle term: it interposed an almost invisible layer of matter between the seer and the seen – the sheen of a window, the silver glaze of the mirror, the convexity or concavity of the lens. (2008, 3)

Armstrong puts forward seven theses about Victorian glassworlds, which are of particular value to the discussion of medical mappings of syphilis. Like modernity, Armstrong postulates, glass is infested with contradictions: conceived in its ever growing purity, it also harbours bodily residues of the workmen who created it. Glass is "an antithetical material" (2008, 11). The breath of the worker, with the minuscule particles of his self, moulds the glass. Translucent, the substance is thus also "stained" by an invisible corporeal film (2008, 4). At the same time, it embodies the lustre, glamour and immense possibility of modern technologies and offers a "glazed urban phantasmagoria [of] reflections" (2008, 8). In this context, not only symbolically but also in a very real sense, glass, as an unsuspected object of transmission, exemplifies the ubiquity, pervasiveness and invisibility of syphilis.

Glass, continues Armstrong, is both a medium and a barrier, which highlights the intricacies of space ownership and by that maps the uneasy relation between the subject and the object (2008, 7). It also, however, marks the times when "spatial boundaries become indeterminate" (2008, 8). In this context, the association of glass and syphilis, both in Philippe's novel and in Western medical writings, marks a moment in time when prophylactic isolationism becomes futile in the combat against the disease. Glass, as a possible, paradoxically pristine, medium of transmission disregards interhuman boundaries and can thus collapse social hierarchies. The scenario of a disease transmitted by the waiter to a middle-class client in a restaurant becomes emblematic. Here, the glass translucence makes evident the necessity of a stringent policing of interpersonal relations while, at the same time, highlighting the futility of preventive projects: if syphilis is paramount and can be transported by means of such pristine objects as glass, how are interhuman relations to be policed?

Syphilis Prophylaxis

In this context, Bulkley regards governmental regulation of prostitution as an inadequate prophylactic measure and calls for a decentralization of responsibility in syphilis prophylaxis. Defining the disease as contagious and making it a criminal offence "would do away with the necessity of officially examining, inspecting, or licensing any one, for it would be for each one's interest to keep free from the disease, lest at any time legal action should be taken against them" (1894, 206). Bulkley has a clear goal in mind: a certification of syphilis as one of the contagious diseases and a concomitant official specification of its treatment and potential penalties in case of transmission (1894, 207). What is characteristic in this case is the elevation of the problem not only to an issue of public health but also to a matter of national security, which, as has been shown, has dominated the perception of the disease for centuries (cf. Pietrzak-Franger 2017, 30–31, 185–231). This uncommon proposal to turn the disease into a case of public offence, which would allow legal measures to be taken against the offenders, however, was impracticable. Bulkley did not manage to outline even a provisionary programme. His absolute belief in the power of law, and disquieting assumption of sufferers' unquestionable compliance, render his argument a case of impractical reveries of wishful thinking.

Bulkley's proposition predated the late nineteenth-century shift from the politics of isolation to the principles of civic responsibility, visible especially in the propositions put forward at the first and second International Conference on Prophylaxis of Syphilis and Venereal Diseases in Brussels (1899, 1902). The 350 governmental and medical members of the congress, representing 33 nations which included Japan, Persia and the United States, consolidated their efforts to combat the disease (1912, 3–4).[12] Under discussion were not only the existing systems of VD control but, most particularly, the recommendations concerning their legal, medical and social regulation. A Berlin physician Dr Blaschko warned against a reductionist, strictly medical approach to the question, proposing to take into consideration "the complex interests of the community – economical, social, ethical" (1912, 6). The proposed prophylactic improvements were concerned either with medical or police supervision or with the question of the legislation of prostitution (1912, 11). While Norway and Spain advised an inspection of all the prisoners rather than only of the prostitutes and while a Bucharest doctor recommended periodical inspection of unmarried men and of pupils in secondary schools as well as of all domestic servants before they enter service, the majority of proposals was "non-coercive" (1912, 16). Such authorities as Fournier and Neisser highlighted the role of knowledge distribution to the combating of the disease. Courses for students and working men, and written notices given to patients were envisaged as adequate means of syphilis prophylaxis. "[P]rotection by knowledge," although clearly gender-specific, was lauded as central to the new methods of syphilis prophylaxis (1912, 16). In an echo strangely evocative of feminist demands concerning women's access to knowledge (see my discussion of Sarah Grand's *Heavenly Twins* and Cicely Hamilton's claims in Pietrzak-Franger 2017, 71–125), the first international congress on syphilis prophylaxis reframed the problem in terms of civic responsibility.

Medical mappings of syphilis made a clear association between venereal syphilis and the centres of modernity. In spatial terms, this involved a hierarchical cartography of syphilis occurrence. Where non-venereal, endemic forms of the disease were only tentatively linked to geographical distinctions while being based on racial peculiarities and class divisions, the spread of its venereal form was considered as tantamount to the degree of the civilizational progress. With the increased emphasis on non-venereal ways of syphilis distribution, the prophylactic emphasis shifted from regulationist attitudes towards an individualized politics of explanation with the promotion of civic responsibility and national accountability as the prospective goal. Writing almost forty years later, Allen Pusey, one of the presidents of the American Dermatological Association, clearly refutes the utility of isolationist measures:

> even if there were not social difficulties which made isolation and quarantine impracticable in syphilis, the number of syphilitics precludes the possibility of using these measures. It is no more practicable to quarantine a half-million of the vigorous adult population than it is, as Burke said, to "draw up an indictment against a whole people." (1933, 94)

The intensification of medical discourses around the non-venereal, extra-genital type of syphilis put forth the ineffectiveness of regulationism as a prophylactic measure and exemplified much broader anxieties concerning the future of the nation. If the disease could be transmitted in a non-venereal way, and if there was no knowing who may or may not have it, how to protect society from this peril? Neither registration of syphilis cases, nor educational or coercive measures, however, seemed to offer a suitable means of syphilis prevention. Activating the vocabulary of civic responsibility, although indicative of changing attitudes towards the illness, was at the same time an expression of helplessness. No practical measures could guarantee a prophylactic success if the disease was prevalent. Even at the time when the virulence of the disease was diminishing, geographical mappings of syphilis continued to spread panic and insist on its ubiquity. As there were no satisfying ways of prophylaxis, medical writings became part of the spatial rhetoric that underwrote diverse and often contradictory discourses concerning the regulation of mobility and its potential role in the spread of venereal diseases.

Notes

1. For further discussion of various geographies of syphilis, see Pietrzak-Franger 2017, 185-231. For the exploration of various regulationist policies in Britain and its colonies, see Walkowitz 1980, Phillips 2006, Howell 2009, Hyam 1990 and Levine 2003.
2. *Preventive Hygiene. An account of the Brussels international conferences 1899 and 1902* notes that, at the first International Conference on Prophylaxis of Syphilis and Venereal Diseases in Brussels (1899), Jonathan Hutchinson presented evidence that syphilis was "steadily diminishing" (1912, 17).
3. Iwan Bloch, who offered a historical taxonomy of syphilis, famously argues in his 1914 paper "The History of Syphilis" that "[e]ach nation [...] named syphilis after the nation or country from which it first received the disease, e.g. – the Indians and Japanese called it the Portuguese; the Russians called it the Polish disease; the Turks, the Frank disease" (1914, 18). See also Pietrzak-Franger 2017, 30–32.
4. It is important to note that out of his 2000 cases, it is 113 that he can with certainty classify as extra-genital, which again gives credence to the small prevalence of *syphilis sinucoitu* (1894, 36). According to him, they constitute around 5.5 per cent of the entire sum of *syphilis insontium* he could observe over the 20 years of his work as a practitioner (1894, 35).
5. There are no clear temporal outlines given, but the sources Bulkley surveyed encompass the period from the early nineteenth century—Mosley, Chelsea, "A Treatise on the Lues Bovilla," 1805—to the end of it, when the publications increased considerably (1894, 335).
6. For details on the history of Poland and its partitions, see Norman Davies 1981, vol. II.
7. Like Cooper, he also envisions prostitution, wars, migration, pilgrimages and commercial trade as offering further dangerous spaces of exchange (Bulkley 1894, 4).

8. On Philippe's work, see Demorest 1956, G. Smith 1950.
9. Syphilis separates [...] it also creates bonds, compassion. If it constitutes an obstacle for Pierre and Berthe's love, it is no less the catalyst of their union. [...] To experience syphilis [and love] together, means to accept life in its ambivalence and in its fullness.
10. For a detailed comparison of French, British and German preoccupations with syphilis, see Schonlau 2005.
11. For a summary of literature on the subject, see Bulkley (1894), 219.
12. The description of the congress, its goals and debates are primarily based on *Preventive Hygiene. An account of the Brussels international conferences 1899 and 1902,* 1912. The pages in brackets reference the pages in this anonymous report.

References

Anonymous. 1912. *Preventive Hygiene. An Account of the Brussels International Conferences 1899 and 1902. By an English Member*. London: John Dale, 1912. 3AMS/E/01. The Women's Library, London.

Armstrong, Isobel. 2008. *Victorian Glassworlds. Glass Culture and the Imagination 1830–1880.* Oxford: Oxford University Press.

Bloch, Iwan. 1914. History of Syphilis. In *A System of Syphilis*, ed. D'Arcy Power and J. Keogh Murphy, vol. 1, 2nd ed., 1–40. London: Frowde.

Bulkley, Duncan L. 1894. *Syphilis in the Innocent (Syphilis Insonitum). Clinically and Historically Considered with a Plan for the Legal Control of the Disease.* New York: Bailey & Fairchild.

Cabanès, Jean-Louis. 1996. Invention(s) de la syphilis. *Romantisme* 26 (94): 88–109.

Clemow, Frank. 1903. *The Geography of Disease*. Cambridge: Cambridge University Press.

Cooper, Alfred. 1895. *Syphilis*. 2nd ed. London: J.&A. Churchill.

Davies, Norman. 1981. *God's Playground: A History of Poland*. Vol. 2. Oxford: Clarendon Press.

Demorest, J.-J. 1956. Le primitivisme de Charles-Louis Philippe. *The French Review* 29 (4): 306–313.

Engelstein, Laura. 1986. Morality and the Wooden Spoon: Russian Doctors View Syphilis, Social Class, and Sexual Behavior, 1890–1905. *The Making of the Modern Body: Sexuality and Society in the Nineteenth Century*. Spec. Issue of *Representations* 14 (Spring): 169–208.

Gilbert, Pamela. 2004. *Mapping the Victorian Social Body*. Albany: State University of New York Press.
Howell, Philip. 2009. *Geographies of Regulation. Policing Prostitution in Nineteenth-Century Britain and the Empire*. Cambridge: Cambridge University Press.
Hutchinson, Jonathan. 1887. *Syphilis*. London: Cassell & Company.
Hyam, Ronald. 1990. *Empire and Sexuality: The British Experience*. Manchester: Manchester University Press.
Levine, Philippa. 2003. *Prostitution, Race and Politics. Policing Venereal Disease in the British Empire*. New York: Routledge.
Nead, Lynda. 2000. *Victorian Babylon: People, Streets and Images in Nineteenth-Century London*. New Haven/London: Yale University Press.
Philippe, Charles-Louis. 1901/2006. *Bubu of Montparnasse*. New York: Shakespeare House.
Phillips, Richard. 2006. *Sex, Politics and Empire. A Postcolonial Geography*. Manchester: Manchester University Press.
Pietrzak-Franger, Monika. 2017. *Syphilis in Victorian Literature and Culture: Medicine, Knowledge and the Spectacle of Victorian Invisibility*. Gewerbestrasse: Palgrave.
Pusey, William Allen. 1933. *The History and Epidemiology of Syphilis*. Springfield: Charles C. Thomas.
Rappaport, Erika. 2001. Travelling in the Lady Guides' London: Consumption, Modernity, and the Fin-de-Siècle Metropolis. In *Meanings of Modernity. Britain from the Late-Victorian Era to World War II*, ed. Martin Daunton and Bernhard Rieger, 25–44. Oxford: Berg.
Schonlau, Anja. 2005. *Syphilis in der Literatur: Über Ästhetik, Moral, Genie und Medizin (1880–2000)*. Würzburg: Königshausen & Neumann.
Sennett, Richard. 1994. *Flesh and Stone. The Body and the City in Western Civilization*. New York/London: W. W. Norton and Company.
Smith, Grover. 1950. Charles-Louis Philippe and T. S. Eliot. *American Literature* 22.3 (3): 254–259.
Smith, Andrew. 2004. *Victorian Demons: Medicine, Masculinity and the Gothic at the Fin-de-Siecle*. Manchester: Manchester University Press.
Snell, Simeon. 1908. Syphilis Communicated by Industrial Implements. *BMJ* 2 (2501): 1678.
Walkowitz, Judith. 1980. *Prostitution and Victorian Society: Women, Class and the State*. Cambridge: Cambridge University Press.
Walkowitz, Judith. 1992. *City of Dreadful Delight. Narratives of Sexual Danger in Late-Victorian London*. Chicago: University of Chicago Press.
Weyl, Thoedor. 1908. *Handbuch der Arbeiterkrankheiten*. Jena: Gustav Fischer.

Stigmatization, Syphilis, and Prostitution: The Discursive Construction of Sex Workers, Disease, and Feeblemindedness

J.L. Schatz

Introduction

The stigmatization of sex work often perpetuates violence toward women through the chastisement of their sexuality regardless of whether they are sex workers. This happens as women are increasingly sexualized in the media in ways that portray them as objects. We can witness this in the case of Belle Knox, who, on revealing she was doing pornography to pay for college, was harassed and threatened in her day-to-day life as a student at Duke University (Knox 2014). These representations can also be seen negatively affecting other women through countless examples of women being sent home from school for dressing too promiscuously, or for "having wanted it" in the case of sexual assault (Bates 2015). At the same time, these sexual stigmatizations help create the very conditions that push many women into prostitution in the first place, because they foreclose other opportunities as a result of sexualized representations that are

J.L. Schatz (✉)
Binghamton University, Binghamton, NY, USA

K. Nixon, L. Servitje (eds.), *Syphilis and Subjectivity*,
https://doi.org/10.1007/978-3-319-66367-8_3

read against the trope of sex work.[1] This is not to say that no women freely choose prostitution. Certainly, Knox chose to go into pornography because it was a means to pay for her education. Rather, it is to say that the women who bear the greatest risk of violence are often the ones least capable of exerting agency to prevent it. To this end, once Knox was identified for her role in pornography she lost the ability to study due to constant death threats and calls to kick her out of Duke. Sadly, her situation is far from the worst manifestation because for many, the conditions start long before they engage in sex work, due to varying socioeconomic factors. No doubt, when race and nationality are taken into account, many women find themselves locked in a cycle that replicates the patriarchal structures that give way to the very stigmatization that pushes women into sex work in the first place.[2] Ultimately, the stigmatization that surrounds prostitution becomes a primary means to police women's sexuality at large by reproducing the worst of the violence and undermining the potential agency that sex work offers as a means of resistance, even for people like Knox.

The demonization of sex work takes on both a moralistic and a utilitarian tone. In the utilitarian sense, sex work becomes a threat via venereal disease as women become the vectors that men must guard themselves against. Internationally, numerous laws target women who engage in prostitution with the responsibility for prevention and testing, despite the fact that the person buying sex is the real risk of transmission (Simowitz 2013). In teen pregnancy education throughout the United States, it is often treated as a woman's responsibility to not dress provocatively in the classroom, or to take the necessary steps to avoid pregnancy, rather than placing that burden equally on men. This hypocrisy can also be seen with Knox, who was demonized for having acted in pornography while the male students who forcefully outed her were not looked down on for having watched it. As a result, when women become the threat of disease due to sex work, and when they are increasingly sexualized, the threat comes to be targeted at all women, who then constantly have their sexuality scrutinized. Even with better education on STDs by "government and NGOs . . . a stigma still prevails in our society . . . [especially with] syphilis . . . [because it] does not show any unique symptom," thereby making all potentially infected people suspect (Anwar 2015).

When these potentially infected people are increasingly associated with sex work, which is connected to any and all women who embrace their sexuality, women themselves become the threat that justifies their policing and demonization in order to protect the rest of the public from the supposed threat they pose. Thus, diseases like syphilis serve as a tangible justification for demonizing sex workers and women, because if society accepts them it could literally mean an end to humanity itself through the spread of disease.

Of course, such utilitarian concerns about STDs do not operate independently of their moralistic counterparts. As with HIV/AIDS, diseases have long been portrayed as just punishments from a higher being against those who sin via sexual promiscuity, even as many religious figures speak out against such hateful discourse (Pieters 1994). This often allows sex workers, homosexuals, and anyone beyond the whitened norm of purity to be grouped into a threatening category that needs to be contained or eradicated to protect the moral order of things. Kamala Kempadoo (1998), an associate professor of women's studies and former sex worker, explains how this has created categories of "good" and "bad" women based on how they exert sexual energy, whether in patriarchal forms of religious monogamy or toward more supposedly rebellious ends that might enable them to live independently. As such, "female sexual acts that serve women's sexual or economic interests are, within the context of masculinist hegemony, dangerous, immoral, perverted, irresponsible and indecent. Construed in this fashion, the image of the whore disciplines and divides women, forcing some to conform to virginity, domesticity and monogamy and demonizing those who transgress these boundaries" (5–6). The very conception of sex work is used to demarcate how sexuality is perceived in the dominant cultural imagination. That imagination is then read onto women regardless of whether they identify as sex workers because the prostitute becomes a stand-in for degeneracy. This is why so many insults hurled at women make reference to their sexuality.[3] In turn, as women are stigmatized further by such insults, they increasingly find themselves at the risk of violence, as in the case of Knox, who was using her sexuality to get the education she needed to live independently. While religion is not always the foremost justification of those who demonize women for their sexuality, the morality opposition to promiscuity that religion provides serves as a backdrop on which such policing is justified legislatively. This is precisely why so many campaigns for legislation against prostitution are spearheaded by the religious right and are often caught up in anti-trafficking discourse and a certain moralism (Bewley 2014).

The surrounding discourse of moralizing sexuality has tangible effects on both sex workers and the larger population that is perceived as sexually indecent. For instance, the belief that sex work is inherently exploitative assumes that women who engage in sex work must have been trafficked; and, by juxtaposition, this suggests those who have not deserved whatever violence they have coming because they should have refused to enter the industry. This results in a savior complex that moralizes female sexuality in order to ensure that "good girls don't go bad." It therefore becomes a legislative and religious imperative to clean up towns and prevent the "girl next door" from turning into how *Playboy* envisions her. As a result, legislatures and anti-sex-work advocates target the assumption that no "real woman" would want to be a prostitute, so the goal should be to save them from the structures of sexualization that put them in that position to begin with. Sadly, "the conceptualization of 'trafficking' influences the understandings of prostitution" so that all prostitution is discursively tied to trafficking because of how it is morally conceived and legislatively enshrined (Lozano 2011, 246). In turn, whether one consented to sex work or not should not be the focal point when asking about prostitution, even if that question is obviously not irrelevant. Rather, the focus must be on the representations that go into what it means to ask any question about consent in the first place. Put simply, a patriarchal society reads individuals as needing to be saved in both cases—either from their own indecency or from threats to their purity. When this happens, women are increasingly limited in their opportunities because they are always already policed into a paradoxical existence in which they should be pure while at the same time being sexually available as objects of consumption.

Contrary to this approach, I contend that by severing the links between prostitution, female victimhood, disease, and sexuality, we can make it possible to forge a new understanding of sex work that goes beyond moralizing tendencies that reproduce violence. Engaging in new understandings is not merely an academic exercise. Rather, it is an exercise that profoundly affects policy solutions. Unfortunately, "because of the heteronormative nature of public morality . . . public spaces are governed by legislation preventing individuals from engaging in acts considered as offensive to those ideals" (Carpenter and Hayes 2014, 158). Therefore, it becomes impossible to merely enter into a legislative conversation without questioning the principles and discourse that form the framework for how the question is approached. Many sex workers, unlike Kempadoo and Knox, never get to have their voices published, go to Duke, or speak at academic conferences. These questions of access, insofar as they are traced back to how ideals for sexual performance operate, require us to examine the discourses that link disease with moral rhetoric and the desire for regulation. In turn, because "policy makers also function within a discursive space that imposes meanings on their world . . . [an] approach that focuses on discursive practices as a unit of analysis can get at how this 'reality' is produced and maintained and . . . [makes] the policy decision in itself . . . a secondary concern" (Doty 1993, 303). Thus, attacking the ideals that surround sexuality is a prerequisite to changing both the laws and the social stigmatization that went into creating them in the first place. Failure to do so ensures those public spaces always violently exclude those who escape the heteronormative social attitudes enshrined in legislation.

Nowhere has this link between the moralizing rhetoric surrounding sex work and the adoption of counterproductive legal solutions been more prevalent than in the case of syphilis. In the early 1900s, the segregation of red light districts in the United States gave way to full-scale prohibition, which gave way to the policing of sexuality at large to prevent the spread of the disease. More recently, similar policies that seek to quarantine red light districts in places like Amsterdam and Nevada have been adopted for the supposed purpose of protecting both sex workers and civil society. In the case of society, by isolating prostitutes away from the majority of public spaces, these policies purport to protect townships from the indecency that supposedly comes with sex work while simultaneously condoning its existence. In the case of prostitutes, such policies are crafted to protect them from violence by supposedly creating a safe space where they can conduct their business with the protection and sanction of government regulation. However, in both cases the policies ultimately fall short because they reproduce the discursive conditions that demonize sex work in the first place by isolating it as a special form of labor needing protection and regulation to prevent the spread of the disease and sexual promiscuity. As a consequence, prostitution continues to be seen as a threat in both body and mind and workers continue to be demonized, even when sex work is legalized. Furthermore, as red light districts isolate prostitution from the rest of the society it becomes increasingly invisible, denying people the knowledge and motivation to actually improve the conditions for those working in the trade.

Paradoxically, even when sex work becomes an accepted reality in legalization schemes, there is almost always a subsequent pushback against its regulation. In turn, even when legalized, sex work is never fully accepted. Instead, such legislative initiatives function as a way to contain sexual depravity in order to produce outlets for it safely away from the rest of the civil society. As a result, campaigns to legalize sex work function in a very similar way to campaigns to criminalize it. The Chicago Vice Commission Report in the 1900s, which "aptly captured the public attitude," had this to say about the subject:

> Prostitution is pregnant with disease, a disease infecting not only the guilty, but contaminating the innocent wife and child in the home with sickening certainty almost inconceivable; a disease to be feared with as great horror as a leprous plague; a disease scattering misery broadcast, and leaving in its wake sterility, insanity, paralysis, the blinded eyes of little babes, the twisted limbs of deformed children, degradation, physical rot and mental decay. (Simowitz 2013, 432)

The fear surrounding the infectiousness of diseases like syphilis thereby increased the fear over moral degeneracy, which came along with looser sexualities tied to sex work. Commissioner Sanger "had been deeply concerned with the problem posed by venereal disease. . . . He was essentially a public health pragmatist . . . [who] transformed the regulation of prostitution . . . [because] syphilis was [perceived as] not just a disease, but also a stand-in for a moral plague" (Simowitz 2013, 432). By looking at how governmental institutions and people take the material reality of STDs like syphilis and problematically graft them onto the social circumstances in which sex workers find themselves in, it is possible to sever falsely drawn links between these disparate concepts that have prevented the adoption of solutions that work. By interrogating the method that goes into status quo policymaking, we can remove the representations that exacerbate such problems and distort even well-intended initiatives. It is syphilis that can provide this stage, because throughout its history, it has been particularly feared among sexually transmitted diseases for its degenerative effects on both the mind and the body.

Morons, Syphilis, and Sex Work

Discourse often resonates more strongly in the popular imagination than even the literal events that inspired it because discourse is the means by which awareness of historical events circulates, and is what enables history to inform the present. In the case of syphilis, no event resonates throughout medical schools and public knowledge more than the Tuskegee experiments (Reverby 2011, 6). In this study, researchers left known cases of syphilis go untreated in black males for forty years in order to learn more about the degenerative effects of the disease. When this came to light in 1972, "it inspired the political push for requirements for informed consent, the protection of vulnerable subjects, and oversight by institutional review boards" (Reverby 2011, 6). However, this push for reform did not effectively change the conditions surrounding the spread of syphilis or the stigmatization of the at-risk populations. Over a decade later, it is now being found out that the John Hopkins University carried out almost identical experiments in the 1940s in Guatemala, where prostitutes were used to infect men to study potential treatments for syphilis (Dance 2015). Again, there was a push for reform, and yet again these initiatives fell short because society placed the blame on the very subjects the scientists were willing to experiment on repeatedly in the name of saving people from the threat of the disease. Consequently, legislation alone can never be the solution because the discourse that frames its target for solving paradoxically enables the conditions for its harms to happen in the first place. This is why even today "for some people . . . the shame of having a sexually transmitted disease can keep them from proactively seeking treatment," even though now there are treatments that can prevent syphilis from progressing (Perkins 2014).

Modern legislation continues this trend in relation to prostitution by emphasizing notions such as "informed consent" that falsely overdetermine the autonomous individual's ability to freely consent to research experiments or sex work. This occurs because "informed consent" is understood to be possible only for people capable of displaying "rationality" on the basis of all available information, which "is considered a neutral act" (Braswell 2011). As such, once individuals give consent to being a test subject or a sex worker, the society all but abandons them to the worst of violence in the name of saving humanity, because people are already irrational if they would consent to this, meaning they lacked autonomy to begin with. Hence, if someone was informed about the indecency of sex work or the risk of syphilis and still consented to participate, then any further moral consideration of that individual would be irrelevant because he or she had already signed that consent and autonomy away. Such overdetermination of the autonomy of informed consent ignores the conditions in which vulnerable populations make the choice to consent in the first place. In short, many people who cannot afford medical treatment, feed their families, or find a place to sleep may consent to experiments and sex work, but that consent is anything but free even if it is informed. In fact, "the socio-economic exclusion of people with disabilities is more likely to put them at risk for exploitation along with, and as sex workers, who may experience exploitation by those who 'purchase' sex and by those who exploit sex workers" (DAWN 2014). If we do not change the discourse through which populations are targeted for syphilis research or for police crackdowns on prostitutions, those populations will miss out on the benefits that any research advancements provide because they will always be the test subjects for the next wave of advancements.

By way of example, the benign neglect of the populations who consent to testing becomes clear when one realizes that, despite being repeatedly targeted for research experiments, black populations receive very few of the benefits of that research and still suffer higher rates of untreated syphilis than whites in America. The self-fulfilling nature becomes obvious because syphilis "is a human disease . . . [but we aren't] getting rid of it . . . [because the] medical approach . . . assumes everyone has equal access to care, which we know isn't true" (NPR 2011). Put simply, the stigmatization of sex workers and the at-risk populations on the basis of race, class, gender, nationality, and sexual identity perpetuates the conditions that leave those populations vulnerable. If blacks and sex workers are perceived as already more likely to have syphilis, researchers will follow that trail and pressure individuals to be exposed to vaccine trials and other experiments for treatments that can be sold to the populations who are less at risk but whose infection more greatly threatens the hegemonic ordering of sexuality.

Of course, the fact that the Tuskegee Study was performed on black people is by no means insignificant. Black male sexuality has long been perceived as threatening, and black female sexuality has been perceived as available and uninhibited. Representations of black sexuality feed on a litany of white fears and taboos: "stereotypes and caricatures of 'black Hottentots' with freakish feminine proportions; of asexual mammies or lascivious Jezebels; of hypersexual black men lusting after white women" (Patton 2012). These fears manifest in scientific classifications that link intelligence with sexuality, morality, and race. Thus,

> research . . . became "a rallying point for eugenicists who predicted doom and lamented our declining intelligence, caused by the unconstrained breeding of the poor and feeble-minded, the spread of Negro blood through miscegenation.["] . . . The category of the moron . . . was a powerful device for drawing a distinction between tainted and pure white people. The formalized understanding of feeblemindedness legitimized white elite fears and eugenic public policies including involuntary sterilization. (Stubblefield 2007, 174–176)[4]

The consequence was that even if white women would consent to having sex with black men, such a decision would be "moronic," proving that the woman was not intelligent enough to know what she was consenting to despite her score on an IQ test. Similarly, the degenerative minds of black men who wished to infect white women with their depraved sexuality started being policed because it was beyond black people's capacity to act civilized, due to feeblemindedness. Syphilis became the connecting point insofar as the initial invisibility of the disease in the mind enabled ramped-up fears of its spreading through the looser sexuality of blackness. This is precisely why the perceived passing and invisibility of mental disabilities that could make one a moron were used to justify expansive regulatory initiatives to weed out anyone feebleminded enough to willingly spread syphilis and miscegenation.[5] In turn, testing syphilis on black men who had sex with prostitutes was only natural because blacks and prostitutes were the very threats that needed to be policed to protect the white, moral majority. In the end, sexuality and disease became a stand-in for intelligence that would remove questions of informed consent from researchers who wanted access to "morons," or black men with syphilis, to study for the greater good of preserving white populations. If blacks and white prostitutes were already morons, they did not have the ability to consent because they were not fully "rational," irrespective of the economic and racialized conditions of the time. Thus, it is no surprise that the majority of the Tuskegee subjects were poor African-Americans, who often could not afford health care, and who thought the tests were designed to help them.

While some might argue that advancements in medicine are available to everyone, the reality is anything but that. It is not just capitalist and imperialist modes of distribution that ensure that only the wealthiest get the best treatments, but also the fact that once populations are determined to be impure, their lives become unworthy of saving altogether. This ideological fact deeply and implicitly affects policymaking, and that in turn determines which groups lack access to medical care and then coerces them to sign up for research experiments. This biopolitical management of populations under the guise of rationality, equal access, and informed consent discounts the relational aspects that make up the self, ignoring the "Foucauldian accounts of the discursive production of the modern individual" that are at play when conceiving of non-ableist formulations of autonomy (Braswell 2011). Quoting Foucault, Ellen Samuels (2014) explains, "This privileging of medical authority in validating identity reflects the modern turn toward visualizing bodies such that 'the 'glance' has simply to exercise its right of origin over truth'" (18). The consequence is a politics of expendability in which whole populations are willingly sacrificed to save those who conform to the dominant society's ideals (Santos 2003). When government policy enters into the mix, it elevates the needs of its citizens above all else, so that the periphery often is not considered at all. Immigrants, foreigners, and populations that do not fit the neat description of what it means to be "American," as defined by those already in power, are left out. This is why a moralized version of Christian purity understands sex as exclusively for reproduction and why it so readily excludes sex workers from the protected purview of the nation-state. Thus, as the threat of syphilis is scientifically attached to sex workers, black people, immigrants, and mentally disabled populations, the ideal of helping the disadvantaged through medical testing or the legalization of sex work is anything but benign because it always happens within a biopolitical discourse that demonizes all those who are different.

Again, it is crucial to realize that the most affected populations are non-white and are considered more prone to sexual promiscuity because they are often the populations that are most at risk in the first place:

> Walter Fernald, superintendent of the Massachusetts School for the Feebleminded, argued in 1918 that "the high-grade [moron] female group is the most dangerous class. . . . They are certain to become sexual offenders and to spread venereal disease or to give birth to degenerate children.["] . . . Terman and his coauthors announced that those who lacked social intelligence should be classified as feebleminded . . . [and that] white women supposedly demonstrated a lack of social intelligence . . . through friendliness with or sexual attraction to black men. (Stubblefield 2007, 177)

Stereotypes of black male sexual desire led to and enabled the Tuskegee experiment in the 1930s, through myths of purity and white female sexuality being threatened by the mental degeneracy of black men. At the same time, they enabled the medical community to justify the forced sterilization of women who transgressed these boundaries to protect civil society (Stubblefield 2007). In total, "32 U.S. states passed sterilization laws between 1907 and 1937" with many of the sterilizations being performed on "mentally ill" or "mentally deficient" individuals (Stern 2016). Many of these laws were modeled on the British Contagious Disease Act, which was passed in the mid-1800s and resulted in the confinement of people found to have syphilis (Jones 2012). In the United States, sterilizing minorities with STDs or people who broke sexual taboos became the recommended treatment, supposedly for the good of the patients, as they would not have the ability to consent to being parents anyway. In fact, many of these laws remained on the books, with sterilization being carried out frequently in minority and disabled populations well into the 1980s (Ko 2016).

The Tuskegee study and the forceful sterilization of sacrificial populations are not isolated incidents. There is a long history of medicine and science willingly sacrificing countless lives for the greater good in order to normalize populations biopolitically. This continues today through bio-certification processes to determine things like who qualifies as disabled and who should be locked away (Samuels 2014, 126). Time and time again in relation to public health, these studies have revolved around both syphilis and sexuality by using one to medically justify the fears about the morality of considering the other. No doubt this can be seen a decade later in the shockingly similar studies carried out by John Hopkins, mentioned previously: "From 1946 to 1948, American public health doctors deliberately infected nearly 700 Guatemalans—prison inmates, mental patients and soldiers—with venereal diseases in what was meant as an effort to test the effectiveness of penicillin. American tax dollars, through the National Institutes of Health, even paid for syphilis infected prostitutes to sleep with prisoners" (McNeal 2010). When inmates failed to contract syphilis from prostitutes, the doctors went as far as to infect them through spinal injections. To be clear, these experiments were not performed out of conscious malice, but in the name of advancing science and medicine. They were done by scientists who believed they were working for the greater good as they went about the banality of their research. And these experiments paved the way for the widespread acceptance today of penicillin saving the lives of those who can afford health care. Yet the benefits of that research still elude the populations it was tested on, as those populations remain a secondary concern and continue to lack adequate access to health care. In short, these studies demonstrate that when researchers approach vulnerable populations, those populations are not their primary concern, because the goals of the research leave those individuals entirely expendable.[6] The prisoners and sex workers were literally written out of existence in the calculation of what was justified in the name of the scientific and medical advancements that were crucial to treating syphilis. Sadly, such advancements ultimately risk magnifying violence because they result in "the collective sacrifice of the periphery [through] . . . a new genocidal and sacrificial illusion, . . . destroying all of humanity in the illusion of saving it" (Santos 2003). Again and again, periods of quarantine (red light districts, hospitals, prisons, national borders) are followed by exclusion and ultimately extermination (criminalization, lack of treatment, forced sterilization, willful infection). In each instance these actions are justified by the stigmatization of vulnerable populations who are always understood as already socially dead.[7]

Again, these examples are by no means aberrations to medical advancement in the war on disease. Rather, they merely highlight

> the atrocious historical entanglement of racism and science, and [illuminate] the continuing medical exploitation of poor people of color. . . . In America today African-Americans remain the least likely demographic to get immunizations of any kind and remain the racial group most likely to have heart disease, diabetes, and other serious illnesses. . . . These experiments . . . [serve] as a further detriment to poor communities as they question the limited medical services available to them. (Sojwal 2008)

Likewise, the populations most likely to engage in sex work and with the least access to medical services remain those in poor and non-white communities, not just in the hallways of Duke.[8] As this happens, whole populations are written off as degenerate and subjected to the worst of industry abuse and governmental policing at the point where they threaten the patriarchal hegemony of a whitened view of sexuality.[9] This is not to say sex work is inherently exploitative, but just that the possibility of exploitation increases as dominant hegemonic norms determine populations to be disposable. A Duke student like Knox certainly experiences more agency in her choice to be in pornography than the sex worker on the streets of Guatemala who agrees to take part in syphilis experiments. At the same time, they are both subject to the violence of a moralizing sexual discourse in both the media and legislation, although to different degrees. As a result, when debates rage about whether prostitution should be legal, they almost always center on how sex workers should be regulated for their own protection or as a guard against disease, without ever taking into account the structural conditions that situate the disparities in medical access. And if not that, they center on the tax benefits of legalization as a way to guard against the evils of the "black market." Neither thesis is "primarily about 'the rights and wrongs of prostitution,' at least not as they are conveyed in the prostitution debate" (Hulusjö 2013, 21). Ultimately, this leads to policy initiatives that continually fail to protect vulnerable populations from exploitation. Rather, our approach to questions of disease and sex work must be "about how women involved in prostitution . . . narrate and make sense of their experiences, and how their narratives and experiences are enabled and constrained by dominant narratives about prostitution" (Hulusjö 2013, 21). Otherwise, the actual populations targeted for saving will have their individual experiences brushed aside by grander narratives of a securitizing medicalization.

Anti-trafficking campaigns are another perfect example of a savior mentality asserting itself both for and against the individuals it wishes to help. It is important to note that trafficking is often perceived as a threat coming from Third World countries, that smuggle otherwise innocent immigrants into the United States or other First World countries.[10] It is also significant that the United States grants protection only to "severe victims of trafficking" through its visa system, with "severe" defined by the will of the district attorney handling the case. Sadly, this has "the unfortunate effect of making eligibility for the T visa dependent upon the victim's capability to assist and cooperate in the prosecution of the trafficker. Ironically, the more severe the trafficking, the more a victim may be psychologically incapable of assisting law enforcement" (Maciel-Matos 2010, 337). In addition, racialized stereotypes all too often come into play when visas are denied to women who might have agreed to sex work or crossed borders illegally but found themselves in horrific conditions that they did not fully agree to: This story "has become familiar through claims by anti-trafficking activists that pimps lure girls into prostitution, then control, exploit, and brutalize them in a manner that renders them akin to slaves," as these narratives are most likely to result in convictions

(Marcus et al. 2014, 225). This is not to criticize district attorneys for cherry-picking their witnesses in order to get a conviction. However, it is to say that "research that depends on such narratives likely paints a skewed picture of the complex environment of prostitution . . . [that] does not allow researchers to independently verify data, understand relevant contexts, observe behavior, or identify changes in subjects' views over time. Such elements are important for understanding prostitution and for developing appropriate policies related to it" (Marcus et al. 2014, 226–27). Until policymakers adopt a more reflexive approach, their solutions will be counterproductive because they will continue to reproduce the problems by presupposing that the populations at the margins of the society are the risks that need to be targeted.

In this way, anti-trafficking legislation like the "Trafficking Protocol" "does not recognize a difference between 'consent' prostitution without slavery and force, and coerced prostitution[, thereby making] the consent of a victim of trafficking . . . irrelevant" (Lozano 2011, 244). As with consent of the feebleminded and that of syphilis test subjects, the consent of trafficking victims' becomes secondary to the illusory benefits of regulating them. Those who would consent are part of the problem, which if accepted could threaten the morality of virginity and patriarchal monogamy. Those who do not consent are part of the moral majority, which then needs to be actively policed to remain pure from those who could degrade it with their depravity or infect it with their venereal diseases. In turn, the response by lawmakers to victims of trafficking by international institutions is to approach them as paradoxically needing to be both saved and eradicated. As a consequence, "the laws that seek to protect women indeed effectively exclude women . . . [through] immigration policies that are increasingly restrictive" (Lozano 2011, 244). Returning to an earlier example, it is not inconsequential that Guatemala is one of the seven countries to which roughly "eighty percent of the [United States] deportees are being sent" when they are kicked out of the United States for violating immigration laws (Cicero-Domínguez 2005, 320). In the end, the state's solution to the problem of vulnerable populations is to further isolate them from negatively influencing the less vulnerable nation-state. Such solutions ignore the fact that it is this very quest to keep others out—whether on the basis of disease, of being "unskilled," or of mental disabilities—that renders populations vulnerable in the first place. Once a population is rendered vulnerable, it is expendable in the name of protecting those less at risk, whose lives are valued more since they are not already socially dead.

To put it in concrete terms, this is why "the trafficking flows within the Americas and the Caribbean follow the general pattern for trafficking worldwide, with victims being trafficked from poorer regions and countries to comparatively richer ones . . . [and] a large proportion of regional victims in the U.S. . . . [coming] from Mexico, Central America, or Caribbean countries" (Kabance 2014, 24). It further explains why the victims of the Guatemala syphilis study withdrew their claims against the United States for damages "after a US District Court ruled the United States was protected under two immunity laws" that denied protection to people overseas (Ruiz-Goriena 2013). It is also why, despite an official apology from President Obama in regard to Guatemala and a commencement speech on racism by Michelle Obama at Tuskegee University, the ongoing legacy of containment, disease, and extermination remains unaddressed. Sex workers, both willing and unwilling, continue to either be criminalized in the United States, and subsequently deported, or absorbed into a legal regime in which the goal is to control their sexuality in order to further a heteronormative agenda. Even "in a system based on [the] legalization . . . [of] prostitution . . . the government may require special registration, licensing, and mandatory health checks that . . . workers have to follow to avoid criminal penalties . . . in order to protect the health and public order" (Day 2012, 156). In doing this, legalization regimes still represent the workers as problems to be dealt with. Hence, it is no surprise that "many women in prostitution feel safer in street prostitution as compared to Nevada brothels . . . [where] prostitutes have little to no control over their 'work' because the individual counties dictate where, when, and to a certain extent, how prostitutes are to perform their services" (Jacobson 2014, 1043). This patriarchal configuration of sex work assumes that the workers themselves are not responsible enough—precisely because they are already irrational enough to engage in sex work—to do so properly. As a result, legalization preserves the stigma associated with prostitution even as it aims to make it acceptable so long as it remains under the state control (Jacobson 2014, 1045). As was the case with red light districts, legalization as a regime helps to establish morally pure spaces that can be protected by isolating locations where sex work can take place under the watchful eye of the government while remaining out of sight. The end point of this process is that sex workers remain overregulated in how they conduct business while at the same time being denied adequate protection from violence because they remain "out of mind" for the dominant society, which believes that the workers deserve whatever happens to them because they freely entered into such a degenerative profession. Thus, prostitutes are stripped of their ability to fully consent and are either regulated to conform to the guidelines that do not have their best interest in mind, or remain criminalized and subject to the expendability of the state. All the while, such a legislation claims to be created for their protection.

Whether it is the effects of syphilis on black people, the sexual depravity of white women who consent to having sex with black men, or criminals trying to skirt immigration procedures, the application of medical models to morality is anything but benign. Nevertheless, such discourses promote themselves as for the good of the prostitute, safer sex, and medical science. However, these very discourses are what create the risk of acute forms of biopolitical violence, insofar as they remain cloaked in moralizing representations of protection. By denying sexual agency to individuals who engage in prostitution, the state seeks to protect its privileged center of citizens with increasingly restrictive regulation of the individual's body and sexuality. As William Haver (1996), professor of comparative literature at Binghamton University, explains,

> At the level of the individual body which is thus exposed in its erotic relations to be primordially political, it has taken the form of a thoroughly moralist discourse on safer sex, a discourse that reveals its essentialist moralism in the concept of the so-called "innocent victim." . . . Above all, there is mounting evidence that this moralist discourse on the clean and proper body simply is not working, either because condoms, dental dams, and clean works for IV drug users are not available, or out of what is called "choice." The logics of separation and containment also operate . . . in the institutional politics of the nation-state, in the nostalgia for a clean and

> proper body politic, in notions of cultural immunity (where cultural community supposedly provides a preemptive cultural immunity), and . . . [wherever] culture is taken to be constituted by race, ethnicity, gender, class, or sexuality. (8)

There is no shortage of examples beyond the few cited in this chapter in which the containment of disease quickly became the containment and extermination of whole populations.[11] What is more important than any individual example is the fact that, much the way syphilis is considered to be prone to spreading through sex, sex too became a disease prone to spreading through degenerative cultural practices brought about by those having sex. As a consequence, protecting the dominant society from the threats posed by these populations functioned in a similar way to inoculating bodies from disease. It became a model of identifying the vectors, eradicating the means of transmission, and controlling those containable elements to create a cure. People were quarantined (through immigration), studied (in syphilis experiments exempted from US law), and left to die until it was considered safe to let some in (those who fit America's perfect idea of what a victim should look like).

Conclusion

The importance of acknowledging how discourses of disease enter the popular imagination is paramount for changing the outcome of the way society deals with the existence of disease and the populations who are most at risk. As recently as 2014, with fears of Ebola outbreaks, American media and political talk was fraught with calls to halt immigration from large parts of Africa and even to criminally charge people for risking exposure to others. However, "using criminal law . . . to punish people for 'spreading disease' is not new. Prostitutes were targeted long before AIDS when the military feared they would infect soldiers with syphilis. . . . What AIDS and Ebola have in common are fear and stigmatization" (Gerber 2014). Hence, it is necessary to find a new discourse for talking about the threat of the disease instead of continually attaching the threat to specific populations, who then become at fault. As long as medicalization is tied up in controlling the spread of degeneracy, which politically comes to be tied up in larger social issues, models of inclusion and exclusion will reproduce counterproductive and increasingly violent outcomes. It is time to recognize empirically "that criminalizing disease in the name of public health . . . does not work" (Gerber 2014).

Moving away from a politics of dignity and respectability is a crucial first step in forming a new language to talk about sex work and syphilis. That means that prior to any policy, individuals should seek to free themselves from the stigmatization attached to diseased, disabled, and sexual bodies. Whether a person is HIV positive, sex positive, citizen negative, or patient zero, the first response must not be fear, containment, and large-scale categorization. To change this, researchers and policymakers should not aim to put these problems out of sight. But unfortunately, "the most common judgments about sex assign dignity to some kinds (married, heterosexual, private, loving), as long as they are out of sight, while all other kinds of sex are no more dignified than defecation in public" (Warner 2000, 36). This is why legislation on gay marriage can be advanced only when the actual object of gay sex remains unseen. Once sex becomes the focal point, the topic loses the respectability of marriage, even though the topic of sex is by no means specific to gay marriage. Instead of focusing on any individual topic concerning sexuality, theorists and politicians would be better off openly interrogating the larger politics surrounding sexuality, free from stigmatizing discourses: "If sex is a kind of indignity, then we're all in it together. And the paradoxical result is that [it is] only when this indignity of sex is spread around the room, leaving no one out, and in fact binding people together, that it begins to resemble the dignity of the human" (Warner 2000, 36). Thus, by embracing indignity and letting go of fears, people can enable a true positivity toward life regardless of how diseased or mentally disabled that life may appear.

Of course, legal questions are intricately bound up with discursive ones, as the law itself operates as a mode of disciplinary discourse. And to be clear, so long as the focus remains on STDs, it is a question that cannot be answered without looking at sexuality, labor, race, and disability in relation to both representations and legislative and medical actions:

> A "sex-positive" approach that values sexual pleasure in itself requires lawmakers and legal scholars to undertake a more honest assessment of what we choose to regulate, what we fail to regulate, and our justifications for these choices. The assumption that sexual pleasure in itself has negligible or negative value is largely unexamined and unchallenged in legal scholarship. . . . Valuing sexual pleasure improves the discourse on what injury the law should permit individuals to consent to for pleasure, sexual or otherwise. (Kaplan 2014, 90–93)

Thus, while many of the harms of the past and the status quo fall on the state's medicalization, we need not retreat from the state or medical models altogether. Rather, we should seek to alter the conditions in which sex and supposedly sexually deranged populations come to be associated with the law and medicine in the first place. The fact that many people do consent to illegal migration, sex work, and medical studies means that one should not deny agency to people who make such choices. Nor should protections for such individuals vanish once they consent, on the grounds that they are too depraved or vulnerable for the state to care about them. By emphasizing a positive relation to sex, sexually transmitted diseases, and degeneracy, law and medicine could change to actually increase the protections most needed by those truly at risk. This change in emphasis would require us to put the discursive dissemination of information before literal contaminations because that is where the prerequisite stigmatization is formed. Once these parameters are changed, atrocities like the Tuskegee Study and the deliberate infection of Guatemalan prisoners and sex workers with syphilis would become unthinkable.

When one looks at populations that are prone to disease, one must not view having disease in a negative light. Disease is a product of social construction just as much as it is a physical reality. It is crucial not to elevate the presence of syphilis to being the entirety of the sex worker who is at risk of contracting it, in the same way it is crucial not to elevate being a sex worker to the entirety of syphilis or the individual. The disease is not what makes them who they are, and who they are is not what makes syphilis what it is. But syphilis is most definitely a part of who they are, and who they are most definitely shapes how syphilis is understood:

> We can therefore no longer think of the future as the restoration of a putatively uncontaminated past. . . . Indeed, safer sex discourse, including not only verbal admonition but an entire range of material and institutional practices, has become an essential part of an entire scientific medical technology of social control such that all illness, disability, and death itself have become essentially moral failings rather than misfortunes. (Haver 1999, 9)

We are all always already both positive and vulnerable. Highlighting certain vulnerabilities and positivities as threatening while isolating certain populations to bear that brunt exacerbates the social conditions that ensure the spread of the disease goes unchecked. Social isolation, rigid medicalization, and extermination ensure that the conditions in poverty-stricken areas will worsen while stigmatized populations will be subjected to increasing violence. Instead, by approaching being positive positively, we can better address the social conditions and circumstances that make being positive or negative a social location to begin with. Only then can the real cure to disease and social isolation be discovered.

Notes

1. It is important to note that not only women end up in sex work. It is also important to note that not all people agree with the either the term 'sex worker' or 'prostitute' because they both carry their own attached stigmas. As a result, I tend to switch between the terms, while acknowledging that no language is perfect in describing the precise nature of everyone in prostitution. In fact, many of the authors quoted in this chapter speak of the growing number of male and transsexual sex workers and actively advocate to see it as a legal form of labor. However, I say 'women' throughout this chapter because the dominant representations of sex work assume the body of a female worker, which many representations then read as a 'prostitute' instead of a 'worker.' In addition, "gender-related claims deserve special treatment because violations of

women's rights are not generally seen as violations of human rights. . . . Because law inadequately deals with the public/private distinction, women's cultural association with home is a major explanatory factor in the failure of the legal regime to protect female migrants from extreme forms of exploitation" (Hartsough 2002, 108).

2. While this point will be returned to, it is worth noting how "the reality is that many women migrate to the United States to work in the sex industry because it offers better opportunities than what is available in their home country. To ignore that reality is harmful to these women. Some feminists argue that describing and portraying the average sex trafficking victim as an 'innocent coerced' undermines the experiences of a large group of women who are not victims but have instead exercised agency in choosing to come to the United States to work the sex industry. This kind of essentialism of what it means to be a sex trafficking victim is harmful because it defines the average victim in such a manner that it necessarily makes all women who choose sex work 'bad' prostitutes who are not worthy of protection. This dichotomy disregards the complexities of sex trafficking and leads to under-certification of trafficking victims" (Rieger 2007, 249).
3. Again, sexual insults are not directed only at women. However, they often rely on the trope of female sexuality to make their point: "This cultural association of power and sex is pervasive throughout our insult vocabulary . . . [in] attempts to hurt other people . . . [through] the language of sexuality. This reveals why sex can be scary, especially for women who are so often positioned as the one who 'gets fucked'" (Wade 2013).
4. It is necessary to point out that Anna Stubblefield herself is at the center of much controversy concerning issues of consent and disability. In 2015, she was convicted of raping a graduate student of hers who had severe disabilities and could communicate only through a practice known as assisted communication. While the graduate student had given consent through this assisted communication, which was the same way he produced all his assignments throughout college, the judge ruled that it was not a legally recognized form of communication for giving consent. As a result, all evidence of this testimony was denied, and for all intents and purposes Stubblefield's graduate student has been deemed legally incapable of ever consenting to sex due to his disability. Meanwhile, Stubblefield has been serving jail time up through the publication of this piece, although her case recently went up for appeal. For more information, see Engber (2015) and McMahan and Singer (2017).

5. As Carlson (2001) further explains, "The dominant patriarchal stereotypes of (white, middle-class) women as passive, vulnerable, procreative vessels were applied to 'feebleminded' women as well, and in fact justified their incarceration. At the same time, the great importance placed on mental ability and 'proper' sexual conduct rendered them invisible, not just insofar as it did not allow them to express their particular perspective, but in the physical sense. The institutionalization of 'feebleminded' women marginalized them, making them completely socially invisible" (128).
6. For the full details on how vulnerable populations have been exploited in the name of syphilis, see Gutmann and Wagner (2011).
7. In relation to social death, Jared Sexton (2011) writes, "In recent years, social death has emerged from a period of latency as a notion useful for the critical theory of racial slavery as a matrix of social, political, and economic relations surviving the nineteenth-century era of abolition, 'a racial calculus and a political arithmetic that were entrenched centuries ago' (Hartman 2007, 6). This "afterlife of slavery," as Saidiya Hartman calls it, challenges practitioners in the field to question the prevailing understanding of a post-emancipation society and to revisit the most basic questions about the structural conditions of antiblackness in the modern world" (22–23).
8. "Sex trafficking could not thrive if women were not systematically oppressed and marginalized. As one author stated: Traffickers successfully lure women into sex work because these women are victims of poverty, of the social practice of marginalizing women, of the failure of some cultures and societies to place a value on traditional women's work, and of the lack of education and employment opportunities for women in developing and transition countries. . . . Around the world, '[w]omen's sexuality is, socially, a thing to be stolen, sold, bought, bartered, or exchanged by others'" (Rieger 2007, 235).
9. "Poverty and unemployment have made many families susceptible to traffickers who prey on their ignorance, lack of education, and lack of economic means. The root causes of trafficking and migration under coercive circumstances share common and overlapping features. Often, violations of women's human rights are the primary causative factor. The failure of the State to respect, protect, and fulfill women's rights can lead to sexual and economic exploitation of women in both public and private spaces. The failure of existing economic, political and social structures to provide equal and just opportunities for women to work has

contributed to the feminization of poverty, which in turn has led to the feminization of migration, as women leave their homes in search of viable economic options [and life opportunities]" (Manjoo 2014, 11).

10. One example of the essentializing tendencies of trafficking is perfectly reflected in the United States' visa system: "Although the T-visa represents an important development . . . it relied on the notion that the problem is 'over there.' So much so that similarly situated domestic victims often did not have access to the same services. All of these laws not only build upon concepts of otherness, but they serve to reinforce the idea that the problem is 'over there' with the Other, and the Self, if at all involved, is so only as 'rescuer'" (Todres 2009, 653–54).
11. Haver (1996) continues, "There have been and, of course, continue to be attempts to sustain the separations of such cultural immunities through a series of institutional practices that function as a kind of cultural inoculation. I am thinking (for example: the list is by no means exhaustive) of U.S. immigration policies (particularly with regard to Haiti), of enforced quarantine of HIV positives (as proposed in the United States and apparently enforced in Cuba), of the refusal of New York State to countenance a needle-exchange program, of proposals for the tattooing, sterilization, and castration of HIV positives, of prison policies, of calls for mandatory testing, and of a blind refusal even to acknowledge that the problem exists. It is in these policies and practices, as well as in the logics of separation and containment that sustain such policies and practices that the AIDS pandemic is in effect genocidal" (8).

References

Anwar, Mohammed. 2015. Combating Syphilis. *The Daily Star*, February 20. http://www.thedailystar.net/combating-syphilis-65465

Bates, Laura. 2015. How School Dress Codes Shame Girls and Perpetuate Rape Culture. *Time*, May 22. http://time.com/3892965/everydaysexism-school-dress-codes-rape-culture/

Bewley, Elizabeth. 2014. A New Form of Ideological Capture: Abortion Politics and the Trafficking Victims Protection Act. *Harvard Law and Policy Review* 8: 229.

Braswell, Harold. 2011. Can There Be a Disability Studies Theory of "End-of-Life Autonomy"? *Disability Studies Quarterly*.

Carlson, Licia. 2001. Cognitive Ableism and Disability Studies: Feminist Reflections on the History of Mental Retardation. *Hypatia* 16(4). http://cr.middlebury.edu/amlit_civ/allen/2012%20backup/vsara/licia-carlson.pdf

Carpenter, Belinda, and Sharon Hayes. 2014. Crimes Again Morality. In *An Introduction to Crime and Criminology*, ed. Hennessey Hayes and Tim Prenzler, 153–166. http://www.academia.edu/215622/Crimes_Against_Morality

Cicero-Domínguez, Salvador. 2005. Assessing the U.S.-Mexico Fight Against Human Trafficking and Smuggling: Unintended Results of U.S. Immigration Policy. *Northwestern Journal of International Human Rights* 4(2). http://scholarlycommons.law.northwestern.edu/cgi/viewcontent.cgi?article=1036&context=njihr

Dance, Scott. 2015. Hopkins Faces $1B Lawsuit over Role in Government Study That Gave Subjects STDs. *The Baltimore Sun*, April 1. http://www.baltimoresun.com/health/bs-hs-hopkins-guatemala-lawsuit-20150401-story.html

DAWN. 2014. *Myths About People with Disabilities and Sexuality Should Not Be Used to Support Legalization of Prostitution.* http://www.dawncanada.net/en-news/myths-about-people-with-disabilities-and-sexuality-should-not/

Day, Kristina. 2012. Addressing the Sex Trafficking Crisis: How Prostitution Laws Can Help. *Creighton International and Comparative Law Journal* 2: 149–172.

Doty, Roxanne. 1993. Foreign Policy as Social Construction: A Post-Positivist Analysis of US Counterinsurgency Policy in the Philippines. *International Studies Quarterly* 37 (3): 297–320.

Engber, Daniel. 2015. The Strange Case of Anna Stubblefield. *The New York Times*, October 25. https://www.nytimes.com/2015/10/25/magazine/the-strange-case-of-anna-stubblefield.html

Gerber, Michael. 2014. Arresting Ebola Carriers Will Not Curb Virus. *Hartford Currant*, October 20. http://www.courant.com/opinion/op-ed/hc-op-gerber-do-not-criminalize-ebola-carriers-102-20141020-story.html

Gutmann, Amy, and James Wagner. 2011. 'Ethically Impossible' STD Research in Guatemala from 1946 to 1948. *Presidential Commission for the Study of Bioethical Issues,* September. http://bioethics.gov/sites/default/files/Ethically-Impossible_PCSBI.pdf

Hartman, Saidiya. 2007. *Scenes of Subjection: Terror, Slavery, and Self-Making in Nineteenth-Century America (Race and American Culture)*. Oxford: Oxford University Press.

Hartsough, Tala. 2002. Asylum for Trafficked Women: Escape Strategies Beyond the T Visa. *Hasting Women's Law Journal* 13: 77–116.

Haver, William. 1996. *The Body of This Death: Historicity and Sociality in the Time of AIDS*. Redwood City: Stanford University Press.

——— 1999. Really Bad Infinities: Queer's Honour and the Pornographic Life. *Parallax* 5(4). https://www.academia.edu/202053/Really_Bad_Infinities_Queer_s_Honour_and_the_Pornographic_Life

Hulusjö, Anna. 2013. *The Multiplicities of Prostitution Experience: Narratives About Power and Resistance*. Malmö University. http://dspace.mah.se/bitstream/handle/2043/16013/2043_16013%20Hulusj%C3%B6%20MUEP.pdf

Jacobson, Brynn. 2014. Addressing the Tension Between the Dual Identities of the American Prostitute: Criminal and Victim; How Problem-Solving Courts Can Help. *Seattle University Law Review* 37: 1023–58. http://digitalcommons.law.seattleu.edu/cgi/viewcontent.cgi?article=2229&context=sulr. 22 May 2015

Jones, Claire. 2012. Prostitution and the Contagious Diseases Acts (1864, 1866 and 1869). *Herstoria,* July 5. http://herstoria.com/prostitution-and-the-contagious-diseases-acts-1864-1866-and-1869/

Kabance, Karie. 2014. The Globalization of Sex Trafficking. *International Affairs: Directed Research Project*, April 29. Washington University in St. Louis. https://ucollege.wustl.edu/files/ucollege/imce/iap.kabance.drp_.pdf. 21 May 2015.

Kaplan, Margo. 2014. Sex-Positive Law. *New York University Law Review* 89: 89–164. Social Science Research Network. http://papers.ssrn.com/sol3/papers.cfm?abstract_id=2308955

Kempadoo, Kamala. 1998. Introduction. In *Global Sex Workers: Rights, Resistance, and Redefinition*, ed. Kamala Kempadoo, and Jo Doezma, 1–27. New York: Routledge.

Knox, Belle. 2014. I'm Finally Revealing My Name and Face as the Duke Porn Star, March 4.

Ko, Lisa. 2016. Unwanted Sterilization and Eugenics Programs in the United States. *PBS*, January 29. http://www.pbs.org/independentlens/blog/unwanted-sterilization-and-eugenics-programs-in-the-united-states/

Lozano, Sandra. 2011. Feminist Debate Around 'Trafficking' in Women for the Purpose of Sexual Exploitation in Prostitution. *Desafíos* 23(1): 217–57. Universidad del Rosario. http://revistas.urosario.edu.co/index.php/desafios/article/download/1617/1445

Maciel-Matos, Enrique. 2010. Beyond the Shackles and Chains of the Middle Passage: Human Trafficking Unveiled. *Scholar: St. Mary's Law Review on Minority Issues* 12 (2): 328–345.

Manjoo, Rashida. 2014. Trafficking of Women: Norms, Realities, and Challenges. *Albany Government Law Review* 7: 5–33. http://www.albanygovernmentlawreview.org/Articles/Vol07_1/7.1.006-Manjoo.pdf

Marcus, Anthony, Amber Horning, Ric Curtis, Jo Sanson, and Efram Thompson. 2014. Conflict and Agency Among Sex Workers and Pimps: A Closer Look at Domestic Minor Sex Trafficking. *The Annals of the American Academy of Political and Social Science* 653 (1): 225–246.

McMahan, Jeff, and Peter Singer. 2017. Who Is the Real Victim in the Anna Stubblefield Case. *The New York Times*, April 3. https://www.nytimes.com/2017/04/03/opinion/who-is-the-victim-in-the-anna-stubblefield-case.html?_r=0. 1.

McNeal, Donald. 2010. U.S. Apologizes for Syphilis Tests in Guatemala. *The New York Times*, October 1. Agricultural Defense Coalition. http://www.agriculturedefensecoalition.org/sites/default/files/file/constitution_1/1J_2010_U.S._Apologizes_for_Syphilis_Tests_on_Guatemalans_1946_1948_Soliders_Prisoners_Mental_Patients_NYTimes_OCT_1_2010.pdf

NPR. 2011. *Science Diction: The Origin of the Word 'Syphilis.'* http://www.npr.org/2011/05/27/136717683/science-diction-the-origin-of-the-word-syphilis

Patton, Stacy. 2012. Who's Afraid of Black Sexuality. *The Chronicle Review*, December 3. http://chronicle.com/article/Whos-Afraid-of-Black/135960

Perkins, Kaley. 2014. Syphilis: Back on the Rise and Still Deadly. *The Guardian*, June 16. http://guardianlv.com/2014/06/syphilis-back-on-the-rise-and-still-deadly/

Pieters, Stephen. 1994. HIV/AIDS: Is It God's Judgment? http://www.thebody.com/content/art5908.html

Reverby, Susan. 2011. 'Normal Exposure' and Inoculation Syphilis: A PHS 'Tuskegee' Doctor in Guatemala, 1946–1948. *Journal of Policy History* 23(1): 6–28. http://journals.cambridge.org/action/displayAbstract?fromPage=online&aid=7974940&fileId=S0898030610000291

Rieger, April. 2007. Missing the Mark: Why the Trafficking Victims Protection Act Fails to Protect Sex Trafficking Victims in the United States. *Harvard Journal of Law & Gender* 30: 231–56. http://www.law.harvard.edu/students/orgs/jlg/vol301/rieger.pdf

Ruiz-Goriena, Romina. 2013. Guatemalan Syphilis Victims Lose Hope in Legal Battle against US. *Christian Science Monitor*, June 14. http://www.csmonitor.com/World/Americas/2013/0614/Guatemalan-syphilis-victims-lose-hope-in-legal-battle-against-US

Samuels, Ellen. 2014. *Fantasies of Identification: Disability, Gender, Race*. New York: New York University Press.

Santos, Boaventura. 2003. Collective Suicide? *Bad Subjects* no. 63. http://bad.eserver.org/issues/2003/63/santos.html

Sexton, Jared. 2011. The Social Life of Social Death: On Afro-Pessimism and Black Optimism. *InTension* no 5. http://www.yorku.ca/intent/issue5/articles/pdfs/jaredsextonarticle.pdf

Simowitz, Aaron. 2013. How Criminal Law Shapes Institutional Structures: A Case Study of American Prostitution. *American Criminal Law Review* 50(1): 417–53. http://papers.ssrn.com/sol3/papers.cfm?abstract_id=1105409

Sojwal, Senti. 2008. Guatamala Syphilis Study: No Isolated Incident. *Pop Dev*. Hampshire College. http://popdev.hampshire.edu/blog/post/guatamala-syphilis-study-no-isolated-incident

Stern, Alexandra. 2016. That Time the United States Sterilized 60,000 of Its Citizens. *Huffington Post*, July 1. http://www.huffingtonpost.com/entry/sterilization-united-states_us_568f35f2e4b0c8beacf68713

Stubblefield, Anna. 2007. 'Beyond the Pale': Tainted Whiteness, Cognitive Disability, and Eugenic Sterilization. *Hypatia* 22 (2): 162–181.

Todres, Jonathan. 2009. Law, Otherness, and Human Trafficking. *Santa Clara Law Review* 49(3): 605–72. http://digitalcommons.law.scu.edu/cgi/viewcontent.cgi?article=1078&context=lawreview

Wade, Lisa. 2013. On the Sexualized Insult (Not for the Faint of Heart). *The Society Pages*, December 29. http://thesocietypages.org/socimages/2013/12/29/on-the-sexualized-insult-not-for-the-faint-of-heart

Warner, Michael. 2000. *The Trouble with Normal: Sex, Politics, and the Ethics of Queer Life*. Cambridge: Harvard University Press.

Marriage, Motherhood and the Future of the Race: Syphilis in Late-Victorian and Edwardian Britain

Joanne Townsend

Speaking during a period when British national identity and its imperial identity were tightly enmeshed, former Prime Minister Lord Rosebery warned Britons that "An Empire is but little use without an Imperial Race" (Smyth 1904, 49). Preserving Britishness and the Empire meant preserving the current and future health of the nation and the British race. Race, in the late-Victorian and Edwardian periods, and in Rosebery's context meant not an articulation of "ethnic difference" but was used "in its early twentieth-century eugenic sense of the 'better breeding' of the British themselves" (Hall 2005, 5). At this time, the Boer War, 1899–1902, presented Britain with the unthinkable: that the British Army could be defeated by a numerically inferior colonial force. This conflict challenged Britain's self-perception as the greatest imperial power in the modern world by revealing not a race of manly heroes like those of popular fic-

J. Townsend (✉)
Independent Scholar, Melbourne, Australia

K. Nixon, L. Servitje (eds.), *Syphilis and Subjectivity*,
https://doi.org/10.1007/978-3-319-66367-8_4

tion, but a recruiting office full of physically substandard defenders of the Empire:

> The facts which came to light during the South African War revealed to us our true position, and the public which had rejoiced vicariously in the triumphs of the heroes of the football field and the cycle track, were dismayed to learn that of those who wished to serve their country in her day of trial a startling number were found physically unfit to carry a rifle, and that even of those who passed the recruiting officer a large proportion were deficient in the physical stamina and the moral qualities which go to make a soldier. (Smyth 1904, 3)

Despite this sort of rather alarmed public perception, most evidence available at the time demonstrated a rise in life expectancy due to the decline in the rates of contagious disease and improvements in healthcare, housing standards and nutrition, and, that people were healthier at the start of the twentieth century than they had been as little as fifty years earlier. Yet, despite these facts, fears about the nation's military capability grew in concert with tensions between the great powers of Europe in the Edwardian period (Macmillan 2014). Britain's next "time of trial" could come at any point as Europe lurched from crisis to crisis, and the experience of the Boer War suggested that the nation would not be physically ready to meet it. Data collected during the recruitment campaigns for the Boer War challenged the muscular Christian stereotype of the Victorian period and revealed that this God not only had feet of clay, but also weak eyes, wheezy lungs and a dicky heart. This *Boy's Own Paper* heroic ideal of British popular culture was revealed for what it was, only ever an empire-building fantasy. The modern army recruit was not one of H. Rider Haggard's gallant imperial adventurers, but a desk-bound clerk, or a factory worker tied to a production line. Evidence showed the overall health was improving, but the anxiety over racial health born in fin-de-siècle narratives of degeneration and exhaustion proved a stronger cultural force than the reality presented by dry scientific data. These fears led in 1904 to the calling of an Inter-Departmental Committee on Physical Deterioration.

Much of the anxiety over British national health in the late-nineteenth and early-twentieth centuries centered around syphilis, that "blot on our civilized life", which was widely identified as a major cause of present racial deterioration and future degeneration by doctors, politicians, and feminists (Richardson 1876, 99). Syphilis became not just a matter of public health, but an urgent national problem. In light of the recruiting crisis, a link was drawn from the substandard diseased recruit back to the unhealthy child he had been, thence to his sickly infancy, and finally to his mother, never quite well since marriage. Dominating this hereditary horror story was syphilis, the "canker...eating away the vitals of the nation" (Pankhurst 1913, 21). The role it played in marriage, motherhood and childhood health became the theme for many politicians, bureaucrats, doctors and feminists in this period. Syphilis was seen as the greatest threat to both the future and the present of the British Empire. It threatened the present through the infection and incapacitation of the armed forces which had, since the Contagious Diseases Acts of the 1860s, been portrayed as particularly vulnerable to this type of contagion. It threatened Britain's future through maternal and congenital infections which would produce a debilitated population incapable of defending its home and empire.

In the 1890s, syphilis became "an obsessive public crisis" and this perception continued through the Edwardian period. It was the explicit or implicit theme of much literature and art, providing "the iconography for stories of the mask, the double, and the shadow" (Showalter 1986, 100). Oscar Wilde's descriptions of the shocking degeneration of the portrait of Dorian Gray, as its subject increasingly descended further into depravity, could be read as the ravages of syphilis on the nation's young men. In Robert Louis Stevenson's (1896) *Dr. Jekyll and Mr. Hyde*, Mr. Hyde, like syphilis, provoked "disgust, loathing and fear" and could have been syphilis personified (1992, 19). H.G. Wells's Morlocks, those "obscene, nocturnal Thing[s]", in his 1895 novel *The Time Machine,* had devolved even further than Stevenson's creation, showing the fate of a degenerate and syphilized Britain (1993, 45–47). The literature of the fin-de-siècle embraced the language of syphilis, creating an aesthetic of infection and degeneration which gave a narrative form to the anxieties of the period.

Popular fiction brought fears of degeneration, dissolution, and disease into the public consciousness. Without even uttering the word syphilis, taboo at the time in this form of narrative, they imaginatively conveyed the potential horrors of racial decline and disturbingly offered a glimpse of an imaginary future populated by the degenerate offspring of the syphilized present.

Recruitment for the Boer War exacerbated fears about degeneracy and national health. Many potential recruits were turned away for failing to meet the Army's physical standards in areas like height and health. These problems, combined with Britain's failure to triumph over what was essentially an amateur army in South Africa, seemed catastrophic in the atmosphere of the impending war dominating national politics. Repeated failures in recruitment and military campaigns were interpreted as an indication of the widespread physical degeneracy of the British people. Britain appeared unready for the war it seemed must inevitably come to Europe in the Edwardian period, and the government determined to identify and remedy the problem before it was too late. Therefore, inspired by the catastrophe of the Boer War, in 1904, the British Government convened an Inter-Departmental Committee on Physical Deterioration which delivered its findings and recommendations later that same year. Such a Committee did not have the weight of a Royal Commission, but did have the advantage of being able to be convened, hear evidence and report more rapidly, thus reflecting the perceived urgency of the situation. This committee's job was to establish a scientific and sociological understanding of the factors causing the physical degeneracy of the British people. The Committee was "[t]o make a preliminary enquiry into the allegations concerning the deterioration of certain classes of the population as shown by the large percentage of rejections for physical causes of recruits for the Army" (1904, v.32, v). The Committee's Report concerned not the men who had been rejected by the armed forces, but the conditions which produced them, and which, if left unameliorated, would continue to produce more such recruits. Future wars and the soldiers who would fight them were its real concern.

The Committee took evidence on a plethora of subjects including the feeding of infants and children, the adulteration of food, housing, alcoholism, domestic science classes for girls, physical education, conditions of employment, working mothers, and venereal disease. It sat for twenty-six days, and in that time examined sixty-eight witnesses, of whom fifty-four were men and fourteen were women. No women were members of the Committee itself, which was composed primarily of officials belonging to the Board of Education. The Committee followed the conventions for taking evidence and interviewing witnesses which had been used throughout the nineteenth century in parliamentary reports. The Report produced attempted to provide a quantitative and qualitative assessment of the lives of the British people, particularly the poor and the working classes, from whom the bulk of military recruits would be drawn. The "officer class" was not of concern here, it was the corps or body of the armed forces, the large mass of men required to fight any war, who were the subjects of the Report. The government wanted to know how to produce the best bodies for conflict, and this Report investigated all influences on that process. Worrying comparisons with Germany drawn in the Report showed Britain's great rival to be more advanced in the social and sanitary sciences, and showing "immense superiority" in urban planning and managing the environment of the modern city (1904, 19). Witnesses called before the Committee were "experts" in the lives of the working classes. Among those called were Charles Booth, the great social cartographer of London, who gave evidence on urban conditions, "Lady Inspectors" of schools and factories, numerous doctors and medical officers, a colonel in the Salvation Army, the presidents of the Royal Colleges of Surgeons of both England and Ireland, and many officials from the armed forces. The Report was a thorough, if not exhaustive, survey of the nation's physical capabilities, and the Committee members hoped that it "will have some effect in allaying the apprehension of who, as it appears on insufficient grounds, have made up their minds that progressive deterioration is to be found amongst the people generally" (92).

The Committee made a number of principal recommendations at the conclusion of the Report. Surveillance of the health and the bodies of the lower classes in particular was one of the strongest recommendations made by the Committee in the pursuit of future racial health and fitness. Their first priority was to recommend that "a permanent Anthropometric Survey…be organised as speedily as possible" (84). The collection of this sort of information, obtained from measuring the heights and weights of elementary school children and factory employees, would provide a set of figures against which to determine if future progress or degeneration had occurred in the national health. The Committee recommended that a "Register of Sickness" be established to account for the presence and progress of all infectious diseases throughout the nation. Through statistics, diseases could be known and better understood than that in the past, particularly syphilis, the only disease to have a section of the Report devoted to it. Keeping an accurate record of this statistical information would clarify whether Britain was fit to maintain her position among imperial powers.

Medical statistics about disease and infection were particularly central to the Committee's work, and here syphilis had a central role. This was even though the statistics given to the Committee by the Army actually showed that syphilis was not a major cause of the rejection of potential recruits. General Sir Frederick Maurice, for many years a General Officer commanding at the military academy Woolwich, had stated in an article published in the *Contemporary Review* that the number of potential recruits rejected on the grounds of infection with all venereal diseases was surprisingly low. He reaffirmed this finding when he was called before the Committee and questioned about the problems of recruiting. Such evidence ran contrary to the general current of belief persistent at the time. Sir William Taylor, the Director General of the Army Medical Service, concurred with General Maurice's views in a very broad sense, but was more hesitant with the regard to the proportions of acquired and inherited syphilis within the Army, and the extent to which this was a cause of physical breakdowns among recruits. Despite the statistics, he affirmed with the general population's anxieties about the state of the Army, Britain's defense and the future of the Empire, remarking "that out of a hundred men who come up willing to be soldiers we have to turn away between 40 and 60 per cent" (Q.155, 6).[1]

The perceived danger of syphilis to marriage, motherhood and children, and thus to the nation meant that it was the very first of the "Special Subjects" which the Committee considered, whatever the statistics showed. Syphilis was, the Committee reported "an active agent in the production of congenital weakness and the degeneracy that accompanies it" (76). Dr. F.W. Mott, physician to the Charing Cross Hospital and pathologist to the asylums of the London County Council, expressed the belief that many deaths due to syphilis were going unrecorded because the disease affected so many different parts of the body that doctors were failing to recognize it as a cause of death (Q. 10472–10477, 382). When asked about syphilis, Dr. Robert Jones described it as "a foul and loathsome disease; it implies a breach of the moral laws, it is indicative of a weakened self-restraint and public knowledge which will cause shame and reproach" (Q. 10891, 399). Yet, despite this sort of evidence and the amount of anxiety surrounding it, the Committee found that there was much less syphilis in the community than even twenty years ago, and that the disease was becoming increasingly less virulent according to a number of witnesses. However, other witnesses like Dr. Frederick Mott and Sir Victor Horsley suggested that statistics on venereal disease were often inaccurate because the shame of the disease often led to under-reporting, therefore, it was difficult to be sure whether the rates of disease were actually decreasing. Scientific discoveries also meant that conditions which had not previously been diagnosed as syphilitic were now being attributed to that disease. Horsley told the Committee that syphilis would often not be listed as a cause of death on a death certificate "because the practitioner under the present system of death certification dare not put it on the certificate because of the prejudice it would incite and for fear of legal action" (Q.10526, 384). Despite problems with reporting, what was apparent was the inadequacy of treatment facilities and programs for those who were infected. The Committee found that there was not enough hospital accommodation to treat venereal diseases, especially for the poorer classes who "do not seem to know the dangers of syphilis" (Q.10467, 382). This was identified as a major problem as it was believed that working-class sufferers were prone to discontinue treatment after the most obvious signs of infection had disappeared, thus increasing the risk of infecting all future sexual partners and passing the disease on congenitally. It raised the specter of ever-increasing numbers of syphilitics going on to infect even more partners and produce more diseased children. The danger of syphilis was deemed so great, the Committee further recommended that a special Commission of Inquiry be established to inquire into "the prevalence and effects of syphilis, having special regard to the possibility of making the disease notifiable and to the adequacy of hospital accommodation for its treatment" (92). Yet, despite that fear of syphilis and the sense of imminent crisis surrounding it, it was not until 1913, as European political crises mounted that a Royal Commission into venereal disease was established.

Sir Alfred Cooper, Vice-President of the Royal College of Surgeons, gave evidence on the subject of syphilis to the Committee. He was a well-known authority on the subject, with numerous publications to his name, and had twice represented Britain at the conferences on venereal diseases held in Brussels in 1899 and 1902. Asked by the Committee if he believed "it to be a national duty to take every possible means to minimize this source of weakness [venereal diseases]", he replied affirmatively (Q. 3830, 164). Cooper agreed with the Committee that the amount and virulence of syphilis had decreased, but undercut his own assertion by painting a frightening picture of the ravages of this disease that confirmed all the fears that the Committee members, the government, the armed forces, and the general public might have had:

> 3818. Will you kindly describe the ravages and complications that ensue from it?—I should place insanity as almost one of the first things—insanity; idiocy; diseases of the bones, producing deformity and disfigurement; diseases of the eyes, producing blindness; diseases of the ear producing deafness; diseases of the internal organs, causing defective nutrition and deficient development; diseases of the nervous system, producing insidious forms of paralysis, locomotor ataxy; and it is responsible for a large proportion of the cases of lunacy and idiocy in our asylums. (Q. 3838, 163)

Cooper's description of the ravages of the disease, with all its attendant imagery of deterioration and degeneration, emphasized why syphilis was of such special interest to the Committee. Syphilis's role in affecting national efficiency was highlighted by Cooper, agreeing with the Committee that Britain's rates of syphilis "compared[d] very unfavourably with those of foreign armies" (Q. 3840, 164). Syphilis gained its prominence in the discourse of national efficiency and fitness, even as infection rates decreased and a more effective treatment, salvarsan, was discovered, because it could affect so many different parts of the body and in so many varied ways. When asked if he believed syphilis to be "one of the chief causes of whatever degeneracy there is?", Cooper replied, "Certainly, the most potent" (Q. 3874, 165).

Responding to the question of whether syphilis was decreasing among London's poor and the lower classes generally, Dr. Eustace Smith, of the East London Children's Hospital, replied that he did not think there was very much less than there had been (Q. 8432, 318). The Committee took a lot of evidence on the subject of venereal disease among the poor, the core/corps of the armed forces. Investigations into the state of the health of poor children were particularly important, as these children would be the ones to fight future wars and be the mothers of generations to come. Dr. James Kerr, Medical Officer to the London School Board, identified syphilis as a major problem among the poor, and reinforced the eugenicism that permeated the Report, stating that many lower-class school children were

> from parents who ought never to have had children. We frequently see feeble-minded mothers coming to school about their defective children, or mothers who tell of feeble-minded husbands loafing at home. Where a perfectly definite cause can be assigned, which is infrequent, syphilis is the most evident. (Q. 776, 40)

Kerr was not inclined to downplay the extent of syphilis in London. He told the Committee that "inherited syphilis is responsible for a much larger amount of gross defects and permanent ill-nutrition among children than can be definitely assigned to it" (Q. 777, 40). Another medical expert called by the Committee, Dr. D.J. Cunningham, Professor of Anatomy at the University of Edinburgh, expressed similar concerns to many of the previous witnesses with regard to syphilis; the problem rendered him almost speechless: "One can hardly use words strong enough about it" (Q. 2216, 97). Dr. Cunningham's special interest was in anthropometrics, and on this basis stated that he believed "that it was a monstrous thing for the State not to take measures to check this most deteriorating disease" (Q. 2216, 97).

In 1907 Britain's first organized eugenics movement, the Eugenics Education Society was founded. This group was small in size, but the language of heredity and evolution was everywhere at this time (Paul

1995, 3).[2] Many people were, to paraphrase Judith Walkowitz, eugenic in their sympathies (1994, 138). They imagined a future in which present problems left unchecked had led to a Britain populated by Wellsian monstrosities and atavistic savages unable to defend its own borders, let alone its imperial possessions. The decreasing virulence of syphilis and modern treatments were also a problem in eugenic terms because, as the Committee on Physical Degeneration suggested, "many syphilitic individuals are preserved to life who are quite capable of reproduction and who, consequently, produce stunted and diseased offspring" (Q. 10532, 384).

Contrary to the widespread public perception of urgent national crisis, and contrary to the tone of the questions asked and answered in their hearings, the Interdepartmental Committee on Physical Deterioration generally found that Britain was not as badly affected by physical degeneration and syphilis as was believed. There had been problems with recruitment in the Boer War, but on the whole the population seemed healthier than it had been in the past. Syphilis had become less virulent and less widespread than it had been. Yet, despite scientific evidence to the contrary, fears about Britain's national fitness and the power of syphilis to undermine the nation continued to be expressed by a variety of groups. The Report acted as a compendium of all the anxieties which preoccupied Edwardian minds. Its moderate conclusions were overwhelmed by the language which surrounded the subject of national health. The lower classes seemed to be in danger of being swept away by the tide of the disease and alcohol brought by modernity. The sexual transmission of syphilis, at the very moment when the conception of a future British soldier or mother might be taking place, along with its hereditary consequences transformed it into a monstrous evil. Syphilis was not just a problem to the present patient, but spread beyond them to affect spouses and children especially. This made it not just a concern for the medical profession, but for many different groups in the British society.

The Report identified maternal health as a key part of improving national health and reducing physical and moral degeneracy. British women played a central role in empire-building though rarely lifting a rifle or mapping new lands. They bore "the burdens of being the mothers of a mighty race, flowing out into all lands to civilize and Christianize, and 'bear the white man's burthen'" (Hall 2005, 33). This "mighty race" had to be healthy and strong enough to conquer both indigenous populations and European rivals. Racial health, and thus maternal health, became a vital part of maintaining the Empire. Girls therefore needed to "take jealous care of their health" (Scharlieb 1895, 6). National health would never improve unless the women who would bear future generations were made aware of the danger syphilis posed to both themselves and their offspring: "It is useless to undertake to solve a question without going to the root of it", A.W. Smyth wrote in 1904, "and the root of national unfitness is the health of mothers during pregnancy" (74). Such concerns were expressed not only by doctors, politicians and bureaucrats, but also by feminists and social purity campaigners. Women needed to be warned about "the rapidity with which physical and mental degeneracy is reducing the most advanced and civilized of peoples like a slowly devouring demon" (Brown 1907, 4). The message that women were the ones who needed to be informed about venereal disease was not new; in the 1860s, the anti-Contagious Diseases Acts campaigners had made the same point, but now it was explicitly linked to the greater imperative of national and imperial progress. For many feminists the answer to this problem lay in the education of women about the perils of marriage and motherhood and how to avoid these potential snares.

By the late-nineteenth century, debates about marriage and motherhood were being couched in increasingly eugenic terms. It was necessary, this argument ran, for women particularly, to make a very careful choice of spouse. Not only did their own health depend on their choice, but so did the future of the nation. As wives they would also be the mothers of the future British race. Women's ovaries were, as Robert Reid Rentoul wrote, "the very birthplace and cradle of the race" (1890, xvi). If they were infected with venereal disease, the consequence would be the production of sickly children. "When you marry", New Woman novelist Sarah Grand warned, "you take the most serious step in life. Not only your own happiness, but the happiness of countless generations depends upon your discretion in the matter" (1898, 96).

The structure and meaning of marriage was a central concern for feminist and social purity campaigners in the later nineteenth century. For the late-Victorian woman, marriage was "perhaps the single most profound and far-reaching institution that would affect the course of her life" (Levine 1989, 150). Statistics showed that between 1871 and 1911 the percentage of women who had ever been married remained between 63.9% and 61% (Lewis 1984, 3). It was one of the most typical of experiences for Englishwomen in this period: "One of the chief stations on this rail in the journey of life" (Butter 1875, 3). The centrality of marriage and motherhood in women's lives was echoed in many feminist texts and speeches in this period. Feminists writing about marriage in the early twentieth century particularly criticized it on economic, social and political grounds. However, it was syphilis and women's sexual ignorance which made the medical aspect of marriage vitally important for many writers on the subject.

Marriage conferred respectability, but it also signified for women the acquisition of sexual knowledge and sexual experience: "Marriage is knowledge, carries knowledge with it", Helena Michie writes, "and not only because of the euphemism that allows us to read knowledge as sex" (2006, 163). Yet, there remained throughout this period, a propensity to see the middle-class wife and mother in this period as "essentially virginal", although the fact of maternity belied a lack of sexual experience (Nelson and Holmes 1997, 2). However, many writers remarked on the ignorance of both single and married women about "the facts of life", particularly of venereal disease. Annie Besant, writing in 1889 remarked on most women's "complete ignorance of their own bodies, which is supposed to be a necessary part of 'female modesty'" (Hall 2005, 32). A contributor to Margaret Llewellyn Davies collection *Maternity* wrote: "I was married at twenty-eight in utter ignorance of the things that most vitally affect a wife and mother" (1978, 44). Those "things" included diseases like syphilis and the effect it had on the health of both women and their children. Dr. Elizabeth Blackwell wrote that education about sex was of such "vital importance to the race" that parents needed to undertake this task very carefully (1882, iii). Feminists pointed out that while most women remained oblivious to the existence of venereal diseases "[m]en already know a great deal, and doctors know most of all" (Pankhurst 1913, 3). Medical texts and journals were full of accounts of women who denied ever having had syphilis, but "had never been really well since her marriage" (Hutchinson 1863, 49–50). These were women who were often ignorant of what made them sick, and unaware of their initial infection.

Women's lack of sexual knowledge was an important and constant theme for British feminists from the nineteenth century onwards. They repeatedly argued that women were deliberately kept in this state of ignorance by the social construction of femininity as an innocent, almost sexless state. In the 1870s, anti-Contagious Diseases Acts campaigner Josephine Butler contended that women needed to know about venereal disease in order to save themselves and their children from contamination. Elizabeth Blackwell, a female physician, warned parents in 1882 that "the adult woman, the center of home influence, must acquire correct knowledge on every subject that concerns family life" (80–1). Sarah Grand made sexual knowledge and ignorance of venereal disease a major theme in her novels of the 1890s, particularly *The Beth Book* and *The Heavenly Twins.*

The campaigners against the Contagious Diseases Acts frequently wrote and spoke about profligate men bringing venereal disease into respectable marriages; a belief reiterated by feminists from this time onwards. Evidence given in the more sensational divorce cases of the period supported their contention by revealing many wives infected by their diseased and dissipated husbands.[3] Medical texts were filled with the stories of women who had unknowingly contracted venereal diseases from their husbands. Louisa Martindale, a surgeon, wrote about a case of a young woman, aged twenty-five, who began experiencing pain and difficulty urinating just two days after her marriage. She came to Martindale with Fallopian tubes inflamed and full of pus, and was "[a]s is usual in such cases…childless" (1908, 26). Her husband later admitted to Martindale that he had contracted gonorrhea prior to his marriage and had also suffered from syphilis, although at the time of his marriage he believed himself cured (1908, 26–27). Doctors Berkeley Hill and Alfred Cooper had noted in 1881 that "the infection of women soon after marriage is an occurrence of considerable frequency" (1881, 391). Women were less likely to be treated for venereal disease, many being kept in ignorance of the nature of their complaint by their husbands: "The husband being very anxious to avoid arousing his wife's suspicions, may allow her, if the symptoms are not troublesome, to go on without advice"

(Hutchinson 1887, 496). Studies of the pregnancies and birth rates of women with syphilis showed patterns of miscarriages and a very high rate of infant mortality. Robert Lee, Assistant-Physician to the Hospital for Children, Great Ormond Street, London described a "family history" of syphilis in an article written for the *British Medical Journal* in 1878: "The *first* child lived one week; the *second* three weeks; the *third* four years; and the *fourth* six weeks" (1878, 820; italics in original). The mother of Edward H., also seen at the Great Ormond Street Hospital, had four healthy children but had had five babies still-born and had miscarried twins (*British Medical Journal* 1880, 205).

Feminists and social purity advocates identified men as the cause of the medical problems of marriage, and particularly the infection of women and children with venereal disease. Man was constructed as licentious and intrinsically unable to be sexually continent. This definition of masculinity as uncontrollably libidinous was made in opposition to the veneration of male chivalry and chastity throughout the nineteenth century arising out of Muscular Christianity. Yet, even texts like Thomas Hughes's *Tom Brown's Schooldays* posited both the heroic virtuous male, Tom Brown, alongside his licentious and "fallen" counterpart, Flashman. For many feminists, far too many men were like Flashman, and not enough were like Tom Brown, and were putting the nation in peril by "constantly infecting and re-infecting the race with vile disease and so bringing about the downfall of the nation!" (Pankhurst 1913, x–xi). Venereal disease became a central trope in the discourse of male immorality and impurity. It was evidence imprinted on the body of a fall from virtue. "We talk of fallen women; but there is never a fallen woman without a fallen man", the Reverend Richard Armstrong wrote, "and often indeed the fall of the man is to a depth far deeper than is hers" (1885, 6). A clear picture of this downward path showed the boy who masturbated and read "vicious" books growing into the man who seduced women, consorted with prostitutes and married and infected his wife with the product of his profligacy, syphilis and produced diseased children "not so much born as damned into the world" (Dyer 1884, 8).

Playwright and novelist Cicely Hamilton saw marriage as the only path manmade society had left open to the majority of women to secure their economic livelihood. Writing in 1909, Hamilton depicted marriage not as the romantic culmination of a woman's life, but "the only means whereby woman, with honesty and honour, shall earn her daily bread" (1981, 36). Hamilton wrote that marriage, as it existed, posed a grave threat to Britain's future not only because of the problems of venereal disease but also because of the narrowness of women's lives and minds. Women were being molded into a "silly angel class", by texts like Edward Hardy's 1892 work *The Five Talents of Women* which narrowly restricted the roles women could fill: "1. To please people. 2. To feed them in dainty ways. 3. To clothe them. 4. To keep them orderly. 5. To teach them" (1892, 129).[4] Such a mentality was forcing women into a "regulation pattern of wifehood:...all home-loving, charming, submissive, industrious, unintelligent, tidy, possessed with a desire to please, well-dressed, jealous of their own sex, self-sacrificing, cowardly, filled with a burning passion for maternity, endowed with a talent for cooking, narrowly uninterested in the world outside their own gates" (1981, 45). Such restrictiveness could only have a negative effect on men as well as women and, she wondered, "what it has meant for the race" (46). She decried the ignorance of women about "certain risks attaching to the state of marriage", and likened the threat posed by syphilis in marriage to the sort of workplace dangers faced by men: "[Y]ou do not, when you turn a man into a pottery or a dynamite factory, sedulously conceal from his the fact that there are such things as lead-poisoning or combustion. On the contrary, you warn him" (46). Yet, too many women were entering marriage entirely unaware of the dangers to themselves and their future children. Those women who did have any sexual and medical knowledge often stumbled on it by accident, much like the heroine of Sarah Grand's *The Beth Book*. Hamilton recounted her own horror on coming across information about syphilis in a book: "we are told we have got to be married, but we are never told *that!*" (55). For this feminist campaigner, syphilis was one of the many issues of which women were kept ignorant by a society that saw her only destiny as wife and mother.

The same qualities Hamilton identified, which she argued women had been taught to regard as making them "good wives", surgeon Louisa Martindale warned also made women easy prey for seducers. Ignorance could lead a woman into prostitution as easily as into marriage. It all depended on the character of the man involved: "She has been taught to be obedient and to be affectionate and charming, and above all to be unselfish. She has been taught to regard her future husband as master, and one she must obey. Surely if she falls into the hands of a scoundrel, there is very little chance that she may successfully resist him" (Martindale 1908, 70). Martindale, echoing the rhetorical framework established by anti-Contagious Diseases Acts campaigners like Josephine Butler, framed her own warning to women about the problems of venereal disease around prostitution and male immorality. *Under the Surface*, published in 1908, had been commissioned by the National Union of Women's Suffrage Societies, and not unnaturally seen the solution to these problems in women winning the right to vote, because "men-made laws are always to the advantage of the man, never the woman" (Martindale 1908, 35). Yet, she too, characteristically in the Edwardian period, also looked to Britain's future, warning that "for the sake of the future sons of England, as well as daughters" issues of prostitution and venereal disease needed to be given vital importance (7).

In response to the "plague" of syphilis in 1913 suffragette Christabel Pankhurst published "one of the period's most hard-hitting attacks on the double moral standard", *The Great Scourge and How to End It* (Bland 1995, 245). Unequivocally, she identified the greatest threat to Britain in the modern period as "[t]he sexual diseases [which] are the great cause of physical, mental and moral degeneracy, and of race suicide" (Pankhurst 1913, vi). Syphilis inextricably linked morality, medicine and racial health for Pankhurst. Her cure for this great evil was twofold, encapsulating the solutions offered by Louisa Martindale and many other feminists into the slogan "Votes for Women and Chastity for Men" (Pankhurst 1913, vii). Syphilis had particular importance for women in determining the nation's present and future health as "[i]t strikes at them in their own person and through their children" (6). For Pankhurst, the interests of women were identical with the interests of the race, and her linking of the issues of racial health and the future of the nation were entirely emblematic of the period. She returned to the issue of race constantly throughout *The Great Scourge*, identifying syphilis as "the prime cause of race degeneration", and darkly noting that if male chastity could not be achieved, then the only way venereal diseases would be eradicated, was by the extermination of the race itself (71, 79). "Votes for Women and Chastity for

Men" were key to the preservation of the British race and nation, as well as central to the feminist campaign for suffrage. She offered her readers a choice of futures. In one, women have won the vote and men have recognized the need to live chastely. Prostitution has disappeared and so has syphilis. Imperial Britain is a healthy nation. In the other future, things have remained unchanged. Britain is faced with "Race Suicide!" (17).

By the Edwardian period, the problems of venereal disease, motherhood, and marriage met in concern for the health and moral well-being of the nation's children who needed to be raised as "manly men and womanly women" (Engstrom 1885, 11). Attitudes to children and childhood had changed quite significantly over the course of the nineteenth century, and childhood was now enshrined as a time of innocence. Children became the "genderless angels'" of the Victorian culture. (Kincaid 1992, 13). This much-cherished ideal was severely tested by the presence of venereal disease, however acquired, in infants and children. Venereal disease represented a threat to both the health of the child and his or her future children and was read as a sign of immorality, if not in the child then in its parents.

There were several ways in which children could become infected with venereal disease. The primary concern in this period was hereditary or congenital syphilis. However, the presence of venereal disease in a child could also be an evidence of sexual assault or abuse.[5] Venereal disease affected children in all classes, although most of the medical records and case studies we possess concern the children of the lower classes, the future soldiers of the British Army, and not those of patients seen in private practice, the officers who would command them. Louisa Martindale stressed that while syphilis appeared to be declining as a cause of infant mortality since 1876, it remained "one of the most active of all maternal infections in the production of congenital weakness and degeneracy in the offspring".[6] The *British Medical Journal* reported in 1895 that 928 out of 1190 males (77.9%) who had died as a result of syphilis in 1893 were under the age of five, as were 745 out of 964 females, or 77.2%, who died of the same cause (*British Medical Journal* 1895, 379–380).[7] These were troubling statistics in a time when it seemed that those children would be needed to defend the Empire and to produce future generations of soldiers.

Doctors writing about children suffering from hereditary syphilis described them as having an unmistakable physical appearance. Syphilis in its congenital form showed itself on the whole body of the child, and often from infancy. In their *Student's Manual of Venereal Disease* Berkeley Hill and Arthur Cooper described the progress of hereditary syphilis in the infant. A baby which may have been born apparently healthy would develop symptoms after two to six weeks. This infant was carefully described for the medical student:

> In a well-marked case the child snuffles as with a cold, is fretful and wastes; by the end of three or four weeks he has generally lost the robust condition he possessed at birth, and gradually gets to look like a little old man; his skin is wrinkled and of a muddy or bistre hue on the forehead, chin and other prominent parts, and often breaks around the mouth, eyes, and nose into chaps that bleed easily. (1886, 46)

Children who survived infancy also showed very characteristic physical signs of congenital syphilis. These children were often characterized as being below weight and height for their ages. They were also identified by "the peculiar condition of the teeth; the thick pasty and greasy skin, especially in the face; the muddy complexion; the sunken bridge of the nose; the scars around the mouth; [and] the prominent forehead" (51).[8] Jonathan Hutchinson, who was the authority on this condition in the late-nineteenth century, described the "prominent frontal eminences like budding horns" of the adolescent syphilitic, providing the demonic alter image of the angelic child of the Victorian fiction (1863, 84). This child was more akin to Wells's Morlocks or Stevenson's Mr. Hyde than to Tom Brown or Alice in Wonderland.

Congenital syphilitic children possessed "a strange uncanny look of age and suffering which is repulsive, and strangely at variance with the cherub-like freshness and innocence of the healthy infant" (Strahan 1892, 152). The presence of congenital syphilis negated childhood as the Victorians understood it:

> There is always an oldness and sedateness about these children, and frequently a characteristic languor. They laugh, but their laughter is like that of grown-up people, it is not the free, happy laughter of childhood. They

> play as if they were playing at play, like old people who play with their grandchildren. (Barraclough 1876, 350)

A baby born with congenital syphilis in Sarah Grand's 1893 New Woman novel *The Heavenly Twins* was despairingly characterized as "old, old already, and exhausted with suffering", and seemingly disturbingly aware of his own unfitness for life, "as his gaze wandered from one to the other it was easy to believe that he was asking each dumbly why had he ever been born" (1992, 289). These children were among the thousands conceived and born each year "with pedigrees which would condemn puppies to the horsepond" (Strahan 1892, 13). A syphilitic child was seen as "a pallid, unhealthy victim of vice for life", and would experience rashes and pains and other health problems, if he survived childhood (A Medical Muser 1888, 593). Even the teeth of these children had a notched, irregular appearance which in connection with other indicators, such as the shape of the skull, were read as an indication of lower evolutionary status.[9] One surgeon remarked that "persons tainted with hereditary syphilis sometimes possess one or more teeth of such magnitude as rather to resemble the tusks of a lower animal than the teeth of a human being" (Barraclough 1876, 350). These children seemed, to their observers, as a long way down the evolutionary scale, and were certainly unfit to take up their duties defending the nation and producing the next generation.

Syphilis played a central role in understandings and representations of Britain's ability to remain one of the world's greatest empires in the late-Victorian and Edwardian periods. Despite statistics which proved the disease was probably less widespread and virulent than it had been only decades ago, syphilis continued to be a matter of obsessive concern in public debates about racial health and deterioration. In 1906, Irish novelist James Joyce wrote: "I presume there are very few mortals in Europe who are not in danger of waking some morning and finding themselves syphilitic" (Hayden 2003, 248). The anxieties it created provided the subtext of much of the science fiction of the period and was the overt concern of New Woman novelists like Sarah Grand. In the first decades of the twentieth century, escalating tensions throughout Europe and Britain's catastrophic defeat in the Boer War drew attention to the health and fitness of the nation's men for armed services. This concern led in

1904 to the Interdepartmental Committee on Physical Deterioration which institutionalized British society's broader panic about this issue, although it had found that statistically syphilis was less of a threat than it had been, and had played little part in the rejection of so many recruits for the South African campaigns. The Committee's Report drew particular attention to the health of mothers and children as the future of British imperial might. Feminist writers in the Edwardian period drew on similar themes by focusing attention on women as the mothers of the race. Syphilis's role in marriage, motherhood and child health became linked to the calls for equal suffrage. "Let all women", Christabel Pankhurst wrote, "who want to see humanity no longer degraded by impure thought and physical disease come into the ranks of the Women's Social and Political Union, and help to win the Vote!" (1913, 145). While more conservative writers might not have agreed with her solution to the problem of syphilis, wider public opinion saw the potential of this disease to destroy Britain's culture, civilization and Empire. What the French writer Guy de Maupassant had earlier described as "[t]he majestic pox, pure and simple; the elegant syphilis" was in the late-Victorian and Edwardian periods "a monstrous evil", an obsessive subject of public concern, given added impetus by the fears of national degeneration and failure it evoked in Great Britain (Quétel 1990, 128–130).

Notes

1. Q. in the citations marks a questions number in the Committee's report and the number that follows indicates the corresponding page.
2. Paul lists the number of members of the British Eugenics Education Society in its first decades as no more than 1200.
3. See Gail Savage (1990). See also Anne Jordan (2010).
4. See also Hamilton (1981, 36).
5. See Jackson (2000) and Taylor (1985, 437).
6. See note in Martindale (1908, 23).
7. The figures from the Registrar-General in 1868 showed that the number of children less than age five whose deaths were attributed to syphilis in that year was, for England and Wales 1472, and for London 386 (Acton 1870, 10).

8. Nancy Stepan has noted the importance given to the skull in racial science as a definition of degenerate types. She writes: "By the late nineteenth century, the urban poor, prostitutes, criminals, and the insane were being constructed as "degenerate types" whose deformed skulls, protruding jaws, and low brain weights marked them as "races apart", interacting with and creating degenerate spaces near at home" (1985, 98).
9. Hutchinson's triad were believed to be the classic indication of hereditary syphilis. The Triad included peculiarly peg-shaped teeth, interstitial keratitis (an affliction of the corneas) and deafness.

References

Acton, William. 1870. *The Contagious Diseases Act. Shall the Contagious Diseases Act Be Applied to the Civil Population?* London: John Churchill & Sons.

Anonymous. 1880. Reports of Medical and Surgical Practice in the Hospitals and Asylums of Great Britain and Ireland. *British Medical Journal*, February 7, 205.

———. 1895. Deaths from Syphilis. *British Medical Journal*, February 16, 379–380.

Armstrong, Richard A. 1885. *Our Duty in the Matter of Social Purity, An Address to Young Men.* London: Social Purity Alliance.

Barraclough, George. 1876. On Hereditary Syphilis and the Contagious Diseases Act. *Medical Times and Gazette*, September 23, 350.

Blackwell, Elizabeth. 1882. *Counsel to Parents on the Moral Education of their Children, in Relation to Sex.* London: Hatchards.

Bland, Lucy. 1995. *Banishing the Beast: English Feminism and Sexual Morality 1885–1914.* London: Penguin.

Brown, Hayden. 1907. *The Wife: Her Book.* London: Sisley's Ltd.

Butter, Henry. 1875. *Marriage for the Millions: For the Lads and Lasses of the Working Classes.* London: W.H. Guest.

Davies, Margaret Llewelyn, ed. (1915) 1978. *Maternity: Letters from Working Women.* London: Virago.

Dyer, Alfred S. 1884. *Facts for Young Men on Moral Purity and Health, Being Plain Words to Young Men upon an Avoided Subject.* London: Dyer Brothers.

Engstrom, C. Lloyd. 1885. *Purity Treated Purely: A Sermon.* London: Rivingtons.

Grand, Sarah. (1893) 1992. *The Heavenly Twins.* Ann Arbor: University of Michigan Press.

———. 1898. *The Modern Man and Maid*. London: Horace Marshall & Son.

H.M.S.O. 1904. *Report of the Inter-Departmental Committee on Physical Deterioration*, 3 vols. London: Dowing & Son.

Hall, Lesley, ed. 2005. *Outspoken Women: An Anthology of Women's Writing on Sex, 1870–1969*. Oxford: Routledge.

Hamilton, Cicely. (1909) 1981. *Marriage as a Trade*. London: The Women's Press.

Hardy, Edward John. 1892. *The Five Talents of Woman: A Book for Girls and Women*. London: T. Fisher Unwin.

Hayden, Deborah. 2003. *Pox: Genius, Madness and the Mysteries of Syphilis*. New York: Basic Books.

Hill, Berkeley. 1881. *Syphilis and Local Contagious Disorders*. London: Smith, Elder.

Hill, Berkeley, and Arthur Cooper. 1886. *The Student's Concise Manual of Venereal Disease: Being a Concise Description of Those Affections and Their Treatment*. London: H.K. Lewis.

Hutchinson, Jonathan. 1863. *A Clinical Memoir of Certain Diseases of the Eye and Ear, Consequent on Inherited Syphilis*. London: John Churchill.

———. 1887. *Syphilis*. London: Cassell & Company.

Jackson, Louise. 2000. *Child Sexual Abuse in Victorian England*. London: Routledge.

Jordan, Anne. 2010. *Love Well the Hour: The Life of Lady Colin Campbell (1857–1911)*. Leicester: Matador.

Kincaid, James R. 1992. *Child-Loving: The Erotic Child and Victorian Culture*. New York: Routledge.

Lee, Robert. 1878. Cases Illustrating the Family History of Syphilis: With Remarks. *British Medical Journal*, June 8, 820.

Levine, Philippa. 1989. 'So Few Prizes and So Many Blanks': Marriage and Feminism in Later Nineteenth-Century England. *Journal of British Studies* 28 (2): 150–174.

Lewis, Jane. 1984. *Women in England 1870–1950*. Hemel Hempstead: Harvester Wheatsheaf.

Macmillan, Margaret. 2014. *The War that Ended Peace: How Europe Abandoned Peace for the First World War*. London: Profile Books.

Martindale, Louisa. 1908. *Under the Surface*. Brighton: Southern Publishing Company.

Medical Muser, A. 1888. The Contagious Diseases Acts. *Lancet,* September 22: 593.

Michie, Helena. 2006. *Victorian Honeymoons: Journeys to the Conjugal.* Cambridge: Cambridge University Press.

Nelson, Claudia, and Ann Sumner Holmes. 1997. Introduction. In *Maternal Instincts: Visions of Motherhood and Sexuality in Britain, 1875–1925*, ed. Claudia Nelson and Ann Sumner Holmes. London: Macmillan.

Pankhurst, Christabel. 1913. *The Great Scourge and How to End It.* London: E. Pankhurst.

Paul, Diane B. 1995. *Controlling Human Heredity: 1865 to the Present.* New Jersey: Humanities Press.

Quétel, Claude. 1990. *History of Syphilis.* Trans. Judith Braddock and Brian Pike. Cambridge: Polity Press.

Rentoul, Robert Reid. 1890. *The Dignity of Women's Health and the Nemesis of Its Neglect.* London: J. & A. Churchill.

Richardson, Benjamin Ward. 1876. *Diseases of Modern Life.* London: Macmillan & Co.

Savage, Gail. 1990. 'The Wilful Communication of a Loathsome Disease': Marital Conflict and Venereal Disease in Victorian England. *Victorian Studies* 34 (1): 35–54.

Scharlieb, Mary. 1895. *A Woman's Words to Women: On the Care of Their Health in England and in India.* London: Swan Sonnenschein.

Showalter, Elaine. 1986. Syphilis, Sexuality, and the Fiction of the Fin de Siècle. In *Sex, Politics, and Science in the Nineteenth-Century Novel*, ed. Ruth Bernard Yeazel. Baltimore: Johns Hopkins University Press.

Smyth, A. Watt. 1904. *Physical Deterioration: Its Causes and Cure.* London: John Murray.

Stepan, Nancy. 1985. Biological Degeneration: Races and Proper Places. In *Degeneration: The Dark Side of Progress*, ed. Edward Chamberlin and Sander L. Gilman. New York: Columbia University Press.

Stevenson, Robert Louis. (1886) 1992. *The Strange Case of Dr. Jekyll and Mr. Hyde*, ed. Emma Lesley. Oxford: Oxford University Press.

Strahan, S.A.K. 1892. *Marriage and Disease: A Study of Heredity and the More Important Family Degenerations.* London: Kegan Paul, Trench, Trübner, & Co.

Taylor, Karen J. 1985. Venereal Disease in Nineteenth-Century Children. *Journal of Psychohistory* 12 (4): 431–463.

Walkowitz, Judith R. 1994. *City of Dreadful Delight: Narratives of Sexual Danger in Late-Victorian London.* London: Virago.

Wells, H.G. (1895) 1993. *The Time Machine*, ed. Michael Moorcock. London: J.M. Dent.

Suspect Bodies, Suspect Milk: Milk Sharing, Wetnursing, and the Specter of Syphilis in the Twenty-First Century

Beatriz M. Reyes-Foster and Shannon K. Carter

Introduction

On a sunny Sunday morning in Orlando, Florida, an infant feeding researcher was making a presentation on breastfeeding. At the end of the presentation, a woman in her 50s rose and thanked her. "I breastfed both of my babies," she explained to the audience, "but having the opportunity to be a wetnurse[1] for a woman in my breastfeeding support group who was sick was the most rewarding experience of my life." The experience she described echoed the findings of our long-term engagement with peer milk-sharing networks in Central Florida. Our interlocutors have often described the experience of milk sharing in highly emotive

B.M. Reyes-Foster (✉)
Department of Anthropology, University of Central Florida,
Orlando, FL, USA

S.K. Carter
Department of Sociology, University of Central Florida,
Orlando, FL, USA

K. Nixon, L. Servitje (eds.), *Syphilis and Subjectivity*,
https://doi.org/10.1007/978-3-319-66367-8_5

terms—one participant who donated anonymously to a local informal milk bank described the feeling on meeting a baby who received breast milk from her as that of "setting [her] heart on fire."

In recent years, peer breast milk sharing[2] has captured the attention of the media as this age-old practice has become more visible due to online social networking. By the same token, the life-saving potential of pasteurized donor milk for medically fragile infants has become increasingly accepted as the Human Milk Banking Association of North America (HMBANA) continues to open and operate non-profit human milk banks in the US and for-profit companies invest millions of dollars in creating breast milk products to market to this population. As these two parallel practices—the direct sharing of breast milk, either in the form of cross-nursing or the gifting of expressed milk, and the biomedicalization of breast milk for use in hospitals—continue to attract attention, old fears and beliefs about breast milk and the women who produce it appear in the guise of new concerns.

While the woman described above spoke of her experience cross-nursing a friend's child in highly positive terms, another woman in the same audience shared that her initial reaction to the thought of feeding her baby another woman's breast milk was largely negative, though on further reflection the thought of acquiring breast milk from a human milk bank seemed reasonable. "Do they screen the milk for diseases in any way? Process it to make sure it is safe?" She asked. This concern with the safety of donor milk, particularly its potential as a vector of disease, is prevalent in social discourses about peer milk sharing. Human milk banks appear to have the ability to symbolically transform suspect breast milk into life-saving "liquid gold" (Carroll 2014).

In this chapter, we consider the contemporary phenomenon of human milk sharing and banking through the parallel lens of nineteenth- and twentieth-century concerns about syphilis and wetnursing. We draw on ethnographic observation, qualitative survey responses, and media representations of peer breast milk sharing to construct our analysis. We identify echoes of earlier concerns with morality and milk in contemporary conversations, noting an interesting contrast between alarmist media representations of peer milk sharing and the way in which milk-sharing mothers understand the risks and realities of peer milk sharing. The notion of trust emerges as an important lynchpin, even when this trust is established in different ways and facilitated by different forms of knowing.

The shadow of venereal disease and its entanglement with notions of morality and cleanliness appears in the form of media representations portraying moral mothers as those whose morality is scientifically proven with rigorous screening—including testing for syphilis. It is also visible in the ways in which peer milk-sharing mothers use other forms of knowing to gauge the trustworthiness of potential donors, specifically in their outright rejection of commodified breast milk. Reminiscent of social attitudes toward wetnurses, who were often seen as lewd and disorderly persons (and who were also uniquely vulnerable to contracting syphilis from their charges), the commodification of breast milk is frequently associated with prostitution and seen as inherently suspect. The intersecting histories of syphilis and wetnursing thus cast a long shadow over breast milk sharing, which occurs in a context informed by this historically situated association between morality and infectious disease.

A Brief History of Syphilis, Breastfeeding, and Wetnursing

Like other venereal diseases, public perceptions of syphilis are entangled with moral judgment. Syphilis was a significant cause of death between the fifteenth and mid-twentieth centuries. Its social stigma has been paralleled to that of AIDS in the twentieth century (Fee 1988). Like HIV, syphilis can be transmitted sexually and non-sexually, yet—also like HIV—it was more frequently associated with immoral behavior. The stigma of syphilis has disproportionately affected women, particularly prostitutes, who have historically been seen as vectors for the disease (Fee 1988; Quetel 1990). Thus, while infants born with congenital syphilis and married women who contracted the disease from their spouses were seen as innocent victims of the disease (Harsin 1989), unmarried women and prostitutes who contracted the illness were subjected at various times to moral hygiene campaigns, social and physical punishment, and incarceration.

The relationship between syphilis and breastfeeding can be traced as far back as the early sixteenth century, when it was discovered that syphilis could be transmitted to a healthy infant by an infected wetnurse, and that healthy wetnurses could be infected by infants born with congenital syphilis (Kertzer 1999, 591). The possibility of an infected wetnurse transmitting the disease to her charge and subsequently the entire family was real (though unlikely) and terrifying. However, although it was rare for a woman with syphilis to transmit the disease to an infant she wetnursed, nearly all healthy women who wetnursed syphilitic infants would acquire the disease and then infect their own families (Harsin 1989; Sherwood 1995). While wetnurses labored under watchful suspicion from their employers, they were far more vulnerable to contracting syphilis from their charges than the other way around.

Historically, women have been the victims of social attitudes and beliefs about syphilis, and this victimization is visible in the history of scientific research on syphilis and breast milk. In eighteenth-century Paris, doctors at the Vaugirard hospital used the bodies of poor syphilitic women as technology to conduct research on treating congenital syphilis in infants. The women were given an aggressive mercury treatment and were then tasked with wetnursing syphilitic infants from an affiliated foundling home (Sherwood 1995, 317). Hailed as one of the first systematic studies of the disease, only 76 children of 407 survived to weaning (332), and the long-term physical and psychological effects suffered by the women who were used in this work remain unknown.

The history of syphilis and breastfeeding must be understood as deeply entangled with the commodification and devaluing of the female body. Just as prostitutes were not only vulnerable to the disease but also to hygiene campaigns and other forms of social stigma, wetnurses were similarly victimized. Like prostitutes, wetnurses were often seen as morally suspect by the doctors and families who hired them. In the nineteenth century, breast milk was not only believed to nourish newborns, but also to pass on moral character, and physicians expressed concern that wetnurses could pass on strange humors into the infants they fed (Sussman 1982). For unwed wetnurses, the fact that they were able to nurse an infant immediately marked them as suspect or immoral (Wolf 1999). Moreover, like prostitutes, wetnurses were vulnerable to contracting the disease from their charges, especially when they were hired to work in hospitals and foundling homes.

Wetnurses, who were of lower social status than the families who hired them, had to contend with ambivalence and "natural repugnance" (Wolf 1999, 101), reportedly experienced by mothers who had to use their services. This repugnance was connected to the perception held by mothers that wetnurses were immoral and qualitatively inferior. Wolf's depiction of wetnursing in Chicago reveals wetnursing as an exploitative profession that frequently led to the demise of wetnurses' own infants. The racial dimensions of wetnursing in the US are also important to take into account. Less than a century earlier, in an activity one hesitates to call "wetnursing" due to the fact that it was forced, uncompensated labor, enslaved women had to nurse their owners' babies at the expense of their own in the antebellum American south (A Negro Nurse 2001).

With the invention of the electric breast pump, breast milk became disconnected from the bodies of women, who no longer had to put nurslings to the breast in order to nourish them. The emergence of biomedical technology that could facilitate the nourishment of infants without the physical presence of a lactating body transformed the nature of human milk. Separated from the body, milk could now become a commodifiable object. At the same time, a gradual shift began taking place away from wetnursing as a profession toward uncompensated milk donation. While twentieth-century physicians believed that breast milk was the perfect food for infants and that access to breast milk could make the difference between life and death, they recognized that hiring a wetnurse could bring significant challenges for employers (Golden 1996). As the development of modern medicine became increasingly scientific, the need to measure and pasteurize donor milk led to the creation of the first Mother's Breast Milk stations around 1910 (Swanson 2011). Rather than personally nurse needy babies, wetnurses could go to the stations, express their milk under medical supervision, and receive payment by the ounce (752). The milk was then blended, pasteurized, bottled, and dispensed.

This shift toward the use of expressed milk coincided with the growing ambivalence toward wetnursing from mothers (Wolf 1999). Hospital-based Mother's Milk stations gave way to milk banks in the 1960s and 1970s, run more like "swaps of outgrown clothes and baby toys." At the same time, a gradual shift began taking place away from wetnursing as a profession towards uncompensated milk donation. Importantly, milk exchanged from these early banks was freely given, not sold. This reverse commodification—from paid wetnursing to free donation—was eventually formalized into the code of ethics of the HMBANA (Lepore 2009). Perhaps in recognition of the exploitative history of wetnursing, HMBANA states in its own position on the ethical allocation of human milk:

> Every infant has a right to be exclusively fed by his or her own mother's milk, and every mother has a right to decide without pressure.…HMBANA does not endorse the practice of selling or purchasing human milk, human milk components, or human milk by-products. (HMBANA n.d.)

Whereas wetnursing was an (often socially stigmatized) occupation, milk donation in the twentieth and twenty-first centuries became an altruistic act. While the HIV epidemic of the 1980s led to the shuttering of the semi-formal milk banks of the 1960s–1970s, HMBANA was established in 1985 to create industry standards for the collection, testing, homogenization, and pasteurization of (uncompensated) donor milk (Swanson 2014). However, although breast milk donors are not compensated for their milk, parents of recipient babies are charged by the ounce for screened and processed human milk.

Today, the sale of breast milk by individuals is often characterized as an entirely different phenomenon to that of formal milk *donation* and even peer-to-peer milk *sharing* (Steube et al. 2014; Reyes-Foster et al. 2015; Palmquist and Doehler 2016).[3] In our research, we have found that women who engage in peer milk sharing reject the notion of being compensated for their breast milk and characterize the sale of breast milk as suspect and immoral (Reyes-Foster and Carter, under review). While wetnursing may have been a stigmatized profession, women who freely donate to milk banks are portrayed in contemporary news media as "lay heroes": altruistic, "kind-hearted" and "generous" mothers (Carter and Reyes-Foster 2016). The shift from suspect paid wetnurses to heroic unpaid milk donors reflects the separation of female bodies from the milk they produce and an interesting transformation in the biovalue of human milk. While the separation of milk from the human body enabled the conditions for its transformation into a commodity, the emergence of biobanking also ensured that human milk's condition as a bodily fluid made it automatically suspect. In her work on biovalue, Catherine Waldby (2002) argues that bodily products–fluids, cells, and tissues-acquire value through their technological processing. Thus, donated blood is suspect and potentially worthless until it acquires biovalue as it is processed into plasma. Thus, as the wet nurse faded into obscurity and bio-banking came into being, human milk came to resemble other types of donated human products. As we have argued elsewhere, (Carter et al. 2015; Carter and Reyes-Foster 2016), the constructed safety of donated breast milk is heavily intertwined with the institutional intervention of the human milk bank, a phenomenon we can identify in other forms of biobanking.

Regarding syphilis, the current biomedical knowledge suggests that it can only be transmitted through breast milk when an active lesion is present on the breast during breastfeeding or breast milk expression (Genc and Ledger 2000; Lamounier et al. 2004; O'Connor et al. 2010). Although several conditions are listed on the US Centers for Disease Control website (CDC 2015) as conditions in which women should avoid breastfeeding, syphilis is not one of them. In a review article of research on syphilis during pregnancy, O'Connor and colleagues (2010, e20) suggest that "Women with syphilis should be advised that breastfeeding is safe for their baby and does not contribute to transmission unless there is a lesion on the breast." The current recommended treatment for breastfeeding mothers with syphilis is to prescribe penicillin and recommend temporary interruption of breastfeeding for 24 hours during the treatment (Lawrence 2013).

There are no published studies that have tested breast milk shared among peers, so there is no way to know for sure whether or not peer milk sharing increases the risk of syphilis transmission. However, individuals who wish to donate milk to milk banks are screened for syphilis, among other infectious diseases including HIV and Hepatitis. Among nearly 2000 potential donors who donated to HMBANA-affiliated milk banks in 2011, 24 (1.2%) were rejected or deferred as a result of any disease infection (Updegrove 2013). A study conducted at the Mothers' Milk Bank of San Jose of 1091 potential donors screened over a six-year period found 0.55% (N = 6) tested positive for syphilis (Cohen et al. 2010). There is no available information on whether or not any of these potential donors had an active lesion on the breast at the time of breast milk expression, which would be required to transmit syphilis from the donating mother to the recipient baby.

Infectious Disease in Milk-Sharing Discourse

Regardless of actual risk of disease transmission through shared breast milk, current media representations present transmission of syphilis and other infectious diseases as a likely outcome of peer breast milk sharing that places innocent babies in immediate danger. In a previous analysis of newspaper articles published in the US between 2010 and 2014 that discuss breast milk sharing, we identified a shift in the characterization of donors and recipients when articles focused on donating and receiving breast milk generally (either through a milk bank or through peers) and sharing breast milk specifically through peers (Carter and Reyes-Foster 2016). In general breast milk donation, infant recipients are portrayed as innocent "victims" who suffer from illness due to prematurity or malnutrition. Breast milk donors are portrayed as lay heroes who altruistically give excess milk that is naturally and abundantly produced by their bodies with little effort. These lay heroes represent the ideal mother due to their dynamic reproductive bodies and their unreciprocated generosity. However, when articles focus specifically on breast milk donation among peers, that is, exchanges that occur outside of milk banks, the narratives of both recipient babies and donors changes. Recipient babies fall victim to the contaminated milk that they receive and peer milk donors become villains who are cast as "bad mothers" who transfer breast milk that is contaminated with disease, harmful substances, or even purposefully diluted for monetary profit.

Throughout the articles, peer-shared milk is presented as a potential vector of the disease, and this risk is suggested to outweigh any potential benefits of feeding a baby breast milk rather than formula. Some articles highlighted the potential for disease transmission in their coverage of official statements by health organizations regarding peer milk sharing, including the following coverage of the US Food and Drug Administration's (USFDA 2015) statement against peer milk sharing.

> *Last week, the agency posted a stern website warning 'against feeding your baby breast milk acquired directly from individuals or through the Internet' because of the danger of infectious diseases and contaminants, including illegal drugs.* (*The Philadelphia Inquirer* 12/7/2010)

Similarly, another article reports that health professionals and the breastfeeding advocacy organization La Leche League International share similar concerns about disease transmission:

> *Still, health professionals and other nursing advocates, including La Leche League International, caution against casual milk sharing because of potential risks to the baby, such as infection, bottle contamination, and the reality that some viruses and diseases are asymptomatic.* (*San Jose Mercury News* 3/29/2011)

Another article discussing a research study that found bacteria in breast milk sold online provides the following "expert testimony":

> *"The study makes you worry," said Dr. Richard A. Polin, the director of neonatology and perinatology at Columbia University, who was not involved in the research. "This is a potential cause of disease. Even with a relative, it's probably not a good idea to share."* (*New York Times* 10/21/2013)

Based on these official recommendations and expert testimonies (Carter and Reyes-Foster 2016), breast milk shared through peer networks is presented as dangerous and risky due to its potential to transmit diseases, including syphilis. Beck (1992) calls western post-industrial societies "risk societies," where the effects of modernization and industrialization are portrayed as growing threats to human health and wellbeing. Risks are not always objective, calculable facts, but instead are socio-historically situated depending on who is considered an "expert." Experts, in turn, reject all risk as acceptable, particularly in the context of bodily fluids–a condition that may well date back to the days when syphilis was a real and prevalent danger.

In contrast to the portrayal of peer breast milk as dangerous, dominant discourses present banked breast milk as safe because of institutional screening and processing (Carter et al. 2015; Carter and Reyes-Foster 2016). Potential donors are tested for a variety of diseases, including syphilis, during the application process to become milk bank donors. The newspaper articles emphasized this screening process in their portrayals of milk banking as safe, which they juxtaposed with peer milk sharing.

> *Health experts encourage mothers—and fathers—to instead [of obtaining milk through the peer milk sharing online network Human Milk 4 Human Babies] get milk from formal milk banks, such as the ones that are a part of the Human Milk Banking Association of North America, a network of nonprofits. Besides being screened for disease, the donated milk is pasteurized before it's made available.* (*Star Tribune* 3/19/2011)

This screening for disease that is required at milk banks, along with processing, testing, and other formalized procedures, contributes to the construction of banked human breast milk as a clean, pure, and sterile substance (Carter et al. 2015; Carter and Reyes-Foster 2016)–an ironic depiction given the fact that milk is an organic and probiotic substance, yet one that is congruent with ideals of scientific mothering.

Whereas some articles referred to "disease" generally, others listed specific diseases for which women who donate milk through milk banks are screened. Syphilis is present on several of these lists, and appears alongside other sexually transmittable infections.

> *Maria DeMarinis Smilios, assistant director of nursing for maternal child services at Flushing Hospital, has been in the health care business for 30 years. She recommends milk banks because they are licensed, and donors are trained with standardized collection and storage techniques. The donors are also tested for transmittable diseases, such as HIV, syphilis and hepatitis, she said.* (*Daily News* 7/28/2011)

> *Milk from a milk bank may reduce some people's trepidation (about our societal fear of germs). Donors are put through rigorous screenings. They must be non-smokers in good health whose blood tests are negative for herpes, HIV and syphilis, Sakamoto said. Their milk arrives to the bank frozen and is thawed, heat-pasteurized to eliminate bacteria, lab tested, frozen and stored before shipment.* (*San Jose Mercury News* 3/29/2011)

Within these portrayals, the screening for disease that takes place at milk banks is presented as a primary mechanism that transforms breast milk from the body of a milk donor from a potential vector of disease to a safe and healthy substance. The appearance of syphilis as one of three potential transmittable diseases listed in the Daily News is particularly notable given the fact the syphilis is not a prevalent illness. The articles list syphilis as a potential threat, and they associate syphilis with HIV, herpes, and hepatitis, thereby emphasizing the sexually transmittable nature of these infections rather than grouping them based on treatability or potential severity. The potential presence or absence of infectious diseases represent within this discourse not only the safety of human breast milk but the purity of the body that produces it. That is, breast milk is only considered safe when it is produced from a maternal body that is perceived as clean—chaste, pure, and scientifically proven to be free from any sexually transmittable infections.

Perceptions of Disease Risk Among Mothers Who Share Milk

Mothers who engage in peer breast milk sharing discuss the possibility of disease transmission through breast milk differently from that which is presented by the news media. In contrast to the alarmist tone present in the news articles, mothers who share milk acknowledge the possibility of disease transmission through shared breast milk, but they portray the risk as small and describe measures they can take to minimize it. As part of our research, we conducted an online survey of about 600 parents who participate in milk sharing. Our survey asked participants to rate peer breast milk, mothers' own milk, and infant formula with regard to health and safety on a scale ranging from very healthy/very safe to very unhealthy/very unsafe. They regarded mother's own milk as the healthiest and the safest, infant formula as the most unhealthy and unsafe, and peer-shared milk as in between the two (Carter, Reyes-Foster and Carter Under Review). In an open-ended question that followed, several participants cited the possibility of disease transmission as a reason they evaluated peer-shared breast milk as less safe/healthy than mothers' own milk. For example, participants stated:

> *There is no guarantee that donor milk was handled properly or that the mother is free of disease.*

> *There is the potential for donor breastmilk to carry disease and thus, potentially be unsafe.*

However, while acknowledging the potential for disease transmission, many participants stated that the risk was small.

> *A donor's milk does carry minimal risk, in my opinion, as it can be a carrier for a few diseases.*

> *Donor milk has a small risk of disease transmission but that risk is small.*

Thus, parents who participate in peer milk sharing are aware of the possibility of disease transmission through breast milk, yet they consider it to be an unlikely occurrence.

Participants also noted that mothers' own milk is a potential vector for disease transmission, and a few attributed an increased risk of disease to infant formula rather than breast milk. Regarding mothers' own milk, many participants stated that it is the healthiest option as long as the mother is free of infectious disease. For example:

> *Mother's milk is always the best thing if she is not infected with a dangerous disease or taking any dangerous medication.*

> *I believe mother's milk to be 100% safe for her baby so long as she is a healthy, drug-free individual who is free of transmittable diseases.*

Some participants suggested that mother's milk was the safest if the mother made responsible feeding choices in relation to her disease status:

> *Mother's milk is the safest as long as the mother is responsible. She knows what disease she has and medications she has taken and can breastfeed or not depending on the safety to her baby.*

With regard to formula, some participants reported its longer-term association with a higher risk of disease as a reason it is less safer than mothers' own or peer-shared breast milk. For example, participants stated:

> *Formula is less safe because of the risks associated with allergies, disease and other illnesses.*

> *Formula raises the risk of a number of complications and diseases over the course of one's life.*

One Participant Simply Stated, *"Formula Causes Disease"*

Many participants described actions that could be taken on the part of breast milk recipients to minimize risks associated with peer breast milk sharing, which overwhelmingly centered on finding a donor they could trust. An important tactic for establishing trust was donor screening. Donor screening was important not only for minimizing risk of infectious disease transmission, but also for assuring the milk was not contaminated with drugs or alcohol, or due to improper milk handling and storage. In an open-ended survey question that asked participants to compare the safety of peer-shared milk with mother's own milk and infant formula, responses like the following were common:

> *Donor breastmilk can be unsafe if you do not know if the donating mother uses drugs or alcohol, has cracked/bleeding nipples and/or disease. If you do your due diligence, I believe it is safe.*

In excerpts like this one, participants acknowledge potential for disease transmission and other risks involved in peer breast milk sharing, and both donors and recipients are responsible for ensuring that donated breast milk is safe. Recipient parents are expected to practice "due diligence" to ensure that their breast milk donors provide milk that is not contaminated with drugs, alcohol, or infectious disease. Recipients are expected to be selective in who they receive milk from by effectively screening potential donors–replicating, in fact, the screening procedures of a milk bank.

For participants in the study, the donor-screening process entailed more than just a checklist of health practices or a review of recent blood work, and was intertwined with the requirement to find a donor they could trust. Overwhelmingly, participants reported that a donor needed to be *trustworthy*—someone who participates in peer milk sharing for the "right" reasons, and therefore would not have a motivation to engage in practices that could jeopardize a recipient baby's health. To be a trustworthy donor, mothers needed to give their breast milk away freely without any expectation of compensation. In a separate survey question, participants drew a sharp distinction between milk sharing and milk selling, describing mothers who sell milk as less trustworthy than those who donate milk. For example, participants stated:

> *People who are selling breast milk probably aren't using as high standards as those who are donating because they are profiting from it.*
>
> *When you buy milk, you run the risk of people adding things to the milk to make more money. That is not the same as meeting a donor in person who gives you the milk out of the goodness of their heart, and who tells you details about their diet.*

This distinction between mothers who donate and those who sell breast milk was echoed in our in-depth interviews with mothers who participate in peer breast milk sharing. Trisha, a 30-year-old white stay-at-home mother who donated milk through peer networks, said:

> *People who are making profit off it, they are trying to pump as fast as they can, they don't really care how they do it whereas we [donors] are trying to help other babies out, are a little more cautious of what we are doing, in my opinion.*

Thus, for our participants, an important aspect of finding a trustworthy donor was to assure that the motivation for donating is to help other babies. This motivation was discerned by a donor giving their breast milk for free rather than receiving any monetary compensation.

Participants expressed that the ability to trust a donor was critical for ensuring that the breast milk obtained through peer networks is healthy and safe to be fed to their babies.

> *Donor milk is safe as long as you can trust the donor to not have been drinking, doing drugs, or have a communicable disease while they were pumping/donating.*

Some participants expressed a need for recipients to get to know their donors in order to establish trust. These discussions relied on a distinction between the known and the unknown: A mother could know the health and safety of her own milk based on the knowledge of her own health behaviors and lifestyle; however, the quality of the milk produced from another woman's body was potentially unknown. By getting to know the donor, a recipient mother should be able to gauge whether or not she can trust that the donating mother's milk is safe.

> *Mom's milk is the safest since she knows what's going into her body. Donor milk is the next best choice, but you have to trust your donor to not have communicable diseases or be on dangerous medications.*

> *Donor milk has risks. If one knows the donor mother, her health and medication history, and trusts her to follow safe storage practices, it is just as safe as mother's milk, but not knowing the donor carries risks of disease transmission, exposure to medications, and improper storage practices.*

For our study participants, trust was critical for assuring that breast milk shared through peer networks was safe. For many, trust was established by getting to know a donor so the recipient could be confident that the donor was free of infectious diseases and avoided practices that could contaminate breast milk such as drug or alcohol use, certain medications, or improper handling and storage.

Overall there is a vast disparity in the dominant discourses of peer breast milk sharing portrayed in news media and those used by mothers who engage in the practice. The dominant discourse uses an alarmist tone to emphasize risk of disease and illness, drawing on broader cultural suspicions of women in general and the female reproductive body in particular. In contrast, mothers who participate in peer breast milk sharing display caution and awareness of risks in their rhetoric; however, they minimize perceptions of risk by emphasizing knowing and trust among the mothers who donate their milk.

Discussion

Both data sets—newspaper discourse showcasing a particular representation of ideal versus suspect donor mothers and open-ended survey responses revealing the importance of establishing trust in milk sharing—present parallel and overlapping concerns about what makes a safe donor, both of which are invested in symbolic notions of cleanliness. In the first instance, scientific measures (rigorous screening, blood work, medical history) ensure that only milk from scientifically clean donors is considered safe for consumption by vulnerable babies. In the second, the gifting of breast milk allows recipient mothers to trust their donors because it disassociates the exchange from prostitution, assuring, again, that the donor mother is clean. In both cases, cleanliness means that donor mothers are free from disease, yet the presence of disease itself is intertwined with notions of female morality that bear a parallel with previous beliefs about wetnurses and their milk.

Two kinds of knowledge converge over a single concern: the morality of mothers who give breast milk. In our analyses of breast milk-sharing discourses in the US news (Carter et al. 2015; Carter and Reyes-Foster 2016), we have argued that news portrayals draw on the idealized image of intensive mothering to portray mothers who give and receive breast milk via formal milk banks as good mothers and those who give and receive through peer networks as bad mothers. Mothers who donate milk to milk banks are portrayed as good mothers as a result of the rigorous screening and training they undergo in order to be approved as donors and because of the altruism inherent in their giving. Mothers who receive milk through milk banks are also presented as moral mothers for using rational decision making in their choice to follow expert recommendations and act in the best interest of their babies. In contrast, mothers who donate milk through peer networks are portrayed as altruistic in their motivations, yet morally suspect because they have not undergone institutional screening and their bodily fluids have not been tested. In these representations, the ability to use scientific testing to prove the purity of the body becomes a marker of the morality of the donating mother. Mothers who receive milk through peer networks are portrayed as morally bad mothers who may be well-intentioned but have not done adequate research about the dangers of peer milk sharing and are consequently exposing their children to unnecessary risk of infection, disease, and even death.

Our analysis in this chapter shows that mothers who participate in peer milk sharing also draw on these hegemonic standards when identifying milk donors who can be trusted to provide safe milk. Participants emphasized that in addition to screening donors, getting to know a donor before accepting their milk was an important precaution that would minimize the risk of infectious disease transmission. Participants reasoned that by getting to know a potential donor's character they could ascertain the safety of the donating mother's milk by determining whether or not they could trust the donor to be honest and to make healthy lifestyle choices. Demonstrating good character requires that potential donors conform to hegemonic standards of mothering. A central tenet to being a trustworthy donor is to engage in unreciprocated giving, which is a key aspect of intensive mothering. An intensive mother is expected to give herself fully to her children, prioritizing them above herself, without any expectation of reciprocation; her fulfillment is actualized in giving to her children (Hays 1996). Similarly, breast milk donors are expected to give their breast milk away freely without any request for compensation. For many donors, the milk is not just stashed in their freezers waiting for a recipient, but is something they actively work to produce and express every day, work that Carroll (2014) identifies as "reproductive labor." However, to request compensation for this labor would call the mother's moral character into question, because, consistent with the intensive mothering ideology, she is expected to be intrinsically fulfilled through giving. The ability to give without considering compensation requires some economic privilege, as milk expression is a time-consuming endeavor that typically involves access to a breast pump and sterile breast milk storage containers. In an online survey of mothers who engage in peer milk sharing throughout the US, Palmquist and Doehler (2014) found that although the participants as a whole were racially and socioeconomically privileged, breast milk donors had slightly higher average incomes than breast milk recipients. The authors conclude that this difference represents the system of "stratified breastfeeding" that operates within the US society, where those of higher socioeconomic status have more resources to invest in breastfeeding, which is also reflected in socioeconomic disparities in breastfeeding rates. Socioeconomic privilege allows breast milk donors to adhere to the principles of intensive mothering through unreciprocated giving because they have the time and resources to express milk to donate to their peers. Mothers who engage in peer breast milk sharing rely on this as a key criterion for identifying trustworthy donors, thereby reinforcing intensive mothering ideologies. Importantly, this perspective was shared by donors and recipients alike.

The notion that the evaluation of a potential donor's breast milk can occur by getting to know their character illuminates the western cultural perception of interconnectedness between bodily purity and morality. The assumption embedded in our participants' narratives is that one's character—what an individual portrays to the outside world—is a reflection of the purity of their body, and hence, an indication of the cleanliness of their milk. This line of thinking is the reverse of what we observed in the dominant discourse portrayed in the US news, yet is another manifestation of the cultural logic that perceives bodily purity and individual morality as intertwined: In the newspaper discourse, bodily purity that could be proven through scientific testing was a marker of a woman's morality. In the mothers' descriptions, a woman's morality as reflected in her character was a marker of her bodily purity.

Conclusion

Syphilis casts a dark shadow in the history of wetnursing that reverberates into contemporary concerns over the morality and trustworthiness of women who donate their milk to human milk banks or to other women. In this chapter, we have described the similarities and differences between two parallel milk donation processes that lead to contrasting socialities. In the first, milk banking, media representations legitimize human milk banks as clean, safe, and stringent. Potential donors must be free of venereal diseases, including syphilis, in what could be seen as much as a measure of morality as of safety. In the second, women recognize the risks of using donor milk and rely on different forms of knowing to determine whether to accept donated breast milk from potential donors. Importantly, in this second process one can observe the emergence of an intimate sociality between donors and recipients based on trust, and the emergence of emotional relationships that imbue gifted milk with deeply emotional value.

In contrast to wetnursing, the reverse commodification of breast milk away from paid work toward a gift economy is facilitating new socialities that stand in contrast to notions of alienation and depersonalization. By the same token, where wetnursing once took place in a context of profound socioeconomic inequality, contemporary milk sharing takes place among peers with significant socioeconomic privilege. This leads to the concern that while poor women no longer have to sacrifice the well-being of their own child for the sake of feeding the child of another in exchange for money, contemporary milk-sharing practices primarily help women who already had the best chances of breastfeeding successfully.

As far removed as contemporary milk sharing appears from syphilis and subjectivity, this chapter demonstrates that many of the same fears and discomforts once associated with syphilis continue to define contemporary concerns and fears about the female body and the life-sustaining sustenance it generates, albeit in different ways. Questions of purity, morality, and the female body are intimately connected to its commodification, and as breast milk shifted from commodity to gift, so has its value.

Notes

1. Although people frequently refer to the nursing of a child by a woman other than the biological mother as "wetnursing," in this chapter *wetnursing* refers to a particular profession that involves compensation. *Cross-nursing* refers to the uncompensated nursing of a child by a woman other than the biological mother. In this particular case, the woman in question was describing her experience of cross-nursing.
2. Peer milk sharing refers to the uncompensated transfer of breast milk from one parent to another. This may be in the form of cross-nursing or in the giving of expressed human milk. In an interesting parallel to the frequent confusion in the use of the term *wetnursing*, human milk sharing is frequently conflated with the sale and purchase of breast milk, though researchers (Stuebe et al. 2014; Reyes-Foster et al. 2015; Palmquist and Doehler 2016) argue the two are separate phenomena.
3. Titmuss (1997) makes a similar argument about gifting versus selling blood.

References

A Negro Nurse. 2001. More Slavery at the South. *The Independent*. New York: Published for the Proprietors, 1848–1921. v. 72, January 25, 1912, 196–200. Retrieved from *Documenting the American South* Electronic Document Depository. http://docsouth.unc.edu/fpn/negnurse/negnurse.html

Beck, Ulrich. 1992. *Risk Society: Towards a New Modernity*. Los Angeles: Sage.

Carroll, Katherine. 2014. Body Dirt or Liquid Gold? How the 'Safety' of Donated Breastmilk is Constructed for Use in Neonatal Intensive Care. *Social Studies of Science* 44 (3): 466–485.

Carter, Shannon K., and Beatriz Reyes-Foster. 2016. Pure Gold for Broken Bodies: Discursive Techniques Constructing Milk Banking and Peer Milk Sharing in U.S. News. *Symbolic Interaction*. Early View: http://onlinelibrary.wiley.com/doi/10.1002/symb.233/abstract

Carter, Shannon K., Beatriz Reyes-Foster, and Tiffany Rogers. 2015. Liquid Gold or Russian Roulette? Risk and Human Milk Sharing in U.S. News. *Health, Risk & Society* 17 (1): 30–45.

Centers for Disease Control and Prevention. 2015. *When Should a Mother Avoid Breastfeeding?* http://www.cdc.gov/breastfeeding/disease/index.htm. Retrieved 6/8/16.

Cohen, Ronald S., Sean C. Xiong, and Pauline Sakamoto. 2010. Retrospective Review of Serological Testing of Potential Human Milk Donors. *Archives of Disease in Childhood-Fetal and Neonatal Edition* 95: F118–F120.

Fee, Elizabeth. 1988. Sin vs. Science: Venereal Disease in Baltimore in the Twentieth Century. *Journal of the History of Medicine and Allied Sciences* 43 (2): 141–164.

Genc, Mehmet, and William J. Ledger. 2000. Syphilis in Pregnancy. *Sexually Transmitted Infections* 76: 73–79.

Golden, Janet. 1996. *A Social History of Wet Nursing in America: From Breast to Bottle*. Cambridge: Cambridge University Press.

Harsin, Jill. 1989. Syphilis, Wives, and Physicians: Medical Ethics and the Family in Late Nineteenth Century France. *French Historical Studies* 16 (1): 72–95.

Hays, Sharon. 1996. *The Cultural Contradictions of Motherhood*. New Haven: Yale University Press.

Human Milk Banking Association of North America (HMBANA). n.d. *Donor Human Milk: Ensuring Safety and Ethical Allocation*. HMBNA Position Paper. https://www.hmbana.org/sites/default/files/images/position-paper-safety-ethical.pdf. Accessed 29 June 2016.

Kertzer, David. 1999. Syphilis, Foundlings, and Wetnurses in Nineteenth Century Italy. *Journal of Social History* 32 (3): 589–602.

Lamounier, Joel A., Zeina S. Moulin, and Cesar C. Xavier. 2004. Recommendations for Breastfeeding during Maternal Infections. *Jornal de Pediatria* 80 (5): S181–S188.

Lawrence, Robert M. 2013. Circumstances when Breastfeeding is Contraindicated. *Pediatric Clinics of North America* 60 (1): 295–318.

Lepore, Jill. 2009. Baby Food: If breast is best, why are women bottling their milk? *The New Yorker*, January 19, New York.

O'Connor, Meghan, Sarah Kleinman, and Meredith Goff. 2010. Syphilis in Pregnancy. *Journal of Midwifery & Women's Health* 53 (3): e17–e21.

Palmquist, Aunchalee, and Kirsten Doehler. 2014. Contextualizing Online Human Milk Sharing: Structural Factors and Lactation Disparity Among Middle Income Women in the US. *Social Science & Medicine* 122: 140–147.

Palmquist, Aunchalee, and Kirsten Doehler. 2016. Human Milk Sharing Practices in the US. *Maternal and Child Nutrition* 12 (2): 278–290.

Quetel, Claude. 1990. *History of Syphilis*. Baltimore: The John Hopkins University Press.

Reyes-Foster, Beatriz, Shannon K. Carter, and Melanie Hinojosa. 2015. Milk Sharing in Practice: A Descriptive Analysis of Peer Breastmilk Sharing. *Breastfeeding Medicine* 10 (5): 263–269.

Reyes-Foster, Beatriz, and Shannon K. Carter. 2018. Mothers, Milk, and Morals: Peer Milk Sharing as Moral Motherwork in Central Florida. In *Breastfeeding: New Anthropological Approaches*, ed. C. Tomori, A.E. Palmquist, and E.A. Quinn. New York: Routgledge.

Sherwood, Joan. 1995. Treating Syphilis: The Wetnurse as Technology in an 18th Century Parisian Hospital. *Journal of the History of Medicine and Allied Sciences* 50 (3): 315–339.

Steube, A., Karleen Gribble, and Aunchalee Palmquist. 2014. Differences Between Online Milk Sales and Peer-to-Peer Milk Sharing. *Pediatrics e-Letter*. Available at http://pediatricsdigest.mobi/content/132/5/e1227/reply

Sussman, George. 1982. *Selling Mother's Milk: The Wetnursing Business in France, 1715–1914*. Chicago: University of Chicago Press.

Swanson, Kara. 2011. Body Banks: A History of Milk Banks, Blood Banks, and Sperm Banks in the United States. *Enterprise & Society* 12 (4): 749–760.

———. 2014. *Banking on the Body: The Market in Blood, Milk, and Sperm in Modern America*. Cambridge: Harvard University Press.

Titmuss, Richard. 1997. *The Gift Relationship: From Blood to Social Policy*. London: London School of Economics.

Updegrove, Kimberly. 2013. Nonprofit Human Milk Banking in the United States. *Journal of Midwifery and Women's Health* 58: 502–508.

U.S. Food and Drug Administration. 2015. *Use of Donor Human Milk*. http://www.fda.gov/ScienceResearch/SpecialTopics/PediatricTherapeuticsResearch/ucm235203.htm

Waldby, Catherine. 2002. Stem Cells, Tissue Cultures and the Production of Biovalue. *Health: An Interdisciplinary Journal for the Social Study of Health, Illness, and Medicine* 6 (3): 305–323.

Wolf, Jacqueline. 1999. 'Mercenary Hirelings' or 'A Great Blessing'?: Doctors' and Mothers' Conflicted Perceptions of Wet Nurses and the Ramifications of Infant Feeding in Chicago, 1871–1961. *Journal of Social History* 33 (1): 97–120.

Part II

Novel Infections

Not-So-Great Expectations: Pregnancy and Syphilis in Sarah Grand's *The Heavenly Twins*

Livia Arndal Woods

> *All [the doctor's] endeavor seems to be not to say what is the matter exactly.*
>
> —Sarah Grand, *The Heavenly Twins*

When Edith Menteith complains to her mother that the doctor treating her mental and physical decline "endeavor[s]…not to say what is the matter exactly," she locates the specificities of her mind and body in unspoken space. Sarah Grand's (1893) *The Heavenly Twins* frames gendered resistance to naming the "exact" "matter[s]" of a lady's venereally disordered body and mind to the lady herself as part a social disease that manifests in dangerous feminine unknowing. And though the novel serves as a particularly pointed *fin-de-siècle* attack on the threats that unsaying and unknowing pose, the narrative nonetheless leaves unnamed the "exact" disease—syphilis—with which Edith's husband has infected

L.A. Woods (✉)
Department of English Language and Literature, University of Michigan, Ann Arbor, MI, USA

K. Nixon, L. Servitje (eds.), *Syphilis and Subjectivity*,
https://doi.org/10.1007/978-3-319-66367-8_6

her. Grand sketches the unspeakable space of syphilis as a large region, extending far beyond what conventional Victorian attitudes about the illness would wish its borders to be. No amount of polite repression, the novel stridently declares, can neutralize the threat this territory poses to futurity: writ on women's reproductive bodies by male licentiousness, syphilis rises up from collective unknowing to trouble the viability of tidy boundaries between mind and body, self and other.

Syphilis is a particular disease, passed between particular bodies in particular ways, that manifests in particular symptoms. Though the particularities of syphilis can vary and though there are vague symptoms associated with the disease—weakness, fever, headache—that can be difficult to diagnose "exactly," there are also distinctive sores, rashes, and patterns of physical and mental deterioration that signal "what is the matter exactly." But the register that can express venereal sores and rashes is resisted in most nineteenth-century fiction in ways that position the particularities of syphilitic bodies in unspeakable space. Not only is somatic specificity resisted in general, but somatic specificity with sexual connotations tends to be especially strongly resisted in Victorian fiction. The Victorian literary tendency to avoid the articulation of sexual somatic particularity also marks tight-lipped narrations of pregnancy in which "all [the] endeavor seems to be not to say what is the matter exactly." Belief in the powers of not saying to effectively repress the influence of transgressive somatic states wears thin at the close of the century, however: fears that unknowing does not protect from the unknown, that the unsaid and unknown particularities of bodies shape futures, and that minds can shape bodies in direct but irrational ways haunt the *fin-de-siècle*.

As somatic states that resist narrative legibility, pregnancy and syphilis in Victorian literature invite critique of the space and work of not saying and not knowing. Maternal impression theory—the theory that what pregnant women see or experience can be reflected in the fetuses they carry—offers a useful lens through which to think about *fin-de-siècle* anxieties about the unspeakable and unknowing agencies of pregnancy and syphilis. This chapter demonstrates that women's reproductive bodies force the revelation of syphilis in *The Heavenly Twins* and frame the novel's deployment of these somatic states in conversation with *fin-de-siècle* anxieties about maternal impression to argue that Grand's novel positions women's bodies as unspeakable sites of unknowing that disrupt futurity through their shaping of children.[1]

Maternal Impression in the *Fin-de-Siècle*

In Thomas Hardy's (1894) *An Imaginative Woman*, a romantic young wife and mother with unfulfilled literary aspirations takes a seaside holiday with her family. There, she learns that she is pregnant with her third child, lawfully begotten of her husband. Ella Marchmill eventually dies giving birth to this child. But, after her death, her husband discovers evidence of her infatuation with a poet, Robert Trewe, whose rooms they had rented at the seaside and whom she never met. Her husband notes a physical resemblance and concludes that his youngest son is the result of a consummated affair:

> When [Ella] had been buried a couple of years it chanced one day that, in turning over some forgotten papers that [her husband] wished to destroy before his second wife entered the house, he lighted on a lock of hair in an envelope, with the photograph of the deceased poet, a date being written on the back in his late wife's hand. It was that of the time they spent at Solentsea.
>
> Marchmill looked long and musingly at the hair and portrait, for something struck him. Fetching the little boy who had been the death of his mother, now a noisy toddler, he took him on his knee, held the lock of hair against the child's head, and set up the photograph on the table behind, so that he could closely compare the features each countenance presented. By a known but inexplicable trick of Nature there were undoubtedly strong traces of resemblance to the man Ella had never seen; the dreamy and peculiar expression of the poet's face sat, as the transmitted idea, upon the child's, and the hair was of the same hue.
>
> "I'm damned if I didn't think so!" murmured Marchmill. "Then she did play me false with that fellow at the lodgings! Let me see: the dates—the second week in August . . . the third week in May. . . . Yes . . . yes. . . . Get away, you poor little brat! You are nothing to me!" (1894, 968)

Marchmill assumes that the resemblance between the poet—now dead—and the boy is a straightforward genetic result of his wife's infidelity. The reader knows that, though Ella had been infatuated with Trewe and dwelt on the idea of him with a sexual intensity during the course of her pregnancy, she never met him, never consummated her feelings, and was already pregnant by the time the fantasy took hold. Indeed, it was as a result of her feeling, upon realizing herself to be pregnant again, that she wished to be "more than a mere multiplier of her kind" that she first began haunting the rooms of Trewe; this is to say, her pregnancy prompts the infatuation, not vice versa as her husband concludes (1894, 956).

In order to confirm his suspicions with the seemingly rationalist evidence of obstetrical science, Marchmill does some hasty math ("let me: the dates—the second week in August…the third week in May…yes…yes"). But in all the punctuation hesitation and grammatically incomplete thought, the reader likely perceives an emptying out of objectivity where objectivity is sought and must accept, instead, that a "known but inexplicable trick of Nature" is responsible for the "strong resemblance" between Ella's child and Trewe. This known but inexplicable trick is maternal impression.

Ann Oakley calls maternal impression a "key theory about pregnancy commonly held prior to the modern obstetric era state[ing] that the condition and viability of the fetus was profoundly influenced by the mother's mental and emotional state" (1985, 23).[2] Cristina Mazzoni calls it "the belief that the fetus can be affected by its mother's desires, fears, [and] experiences" (2002, ix), and Philip Wilson calls it "an age-old belief, which persists in many cultures, [and] alleges that a pregnant woman's imagination, frights, or longings can be transferred to her unborn child, thereby imprinting the child with characteristic marks or deformities." Wilson offers the literary and cultural instances of, for example, a "strawberry-shaped birthmark" understood to result from a pregnant-craving for strawberries, a leech marking on the child of a woman who was bleeding with a particularly large leech during pregnancy, and "a child's resemblance to either parent" (2002, 2). This is to say that maternal impression is associated with pregnancy-cravings, with strong fears and emotions experienced during pregnancy, and with a mother's looking with strong feeling at herself or her spouse during pregnancy.[3]

Maternal impression theories regarding the connection of body and mind during pregnancy specifically were particularly prevalent during the Renaissance and sustained themselves through the medical and scientific revolutions of the Enlightenment. Though there was some "lively intellectual debate" during the eighteenth century as to whether or not the kinds of markings and "monstrosities" that had hitherto been ascribed to maternal imagination were indeed a result of cravings and scares in pregnancy, creative literature of that period frequently and uncritically engages with notions of maternal impression (16). Philip Wilson (2002) notes the deployment of maternal impression, for example, in the novels of Henry Fielding, Lawrence Stern, and Tobias Smollett.[4]

Literary and serious scientific treatments of maternal impression theory, however, recede from view for much of the mid- and late nineteenth century, along with frank representations of sexuality and pregnancy more generally. As women's reproductive lives fell under increasing medical controls, ascriptions of pregnant agency shifted from female minds and bodies to masculine expertise. Maternal impression theory became a mainstay of the circus freak-show tale rather than literary realism. However, at the *fin-de-siècle* when pregnancy re-appears as something more than just the narrative moral lesson it has been for most of the century prior, impression theories seem to re-appear alongside it, even though rationalist belief in maternal impression is no longer prevalent. The deployment of outdated theory in *fin-de-siècle* fiction suggests that notions of impression are *doing something* in late-Victorian fiction, specifically acting as a way of sketching the unarticulated spaces of women's bodies and minds in order to express rising unease with the disruptive social and physical potential of the unconscious mind.

Maternal impression is invoked to make sense of Ella Marchmill's son's resemblance to Trewe in Hardy's story: Ella craves contact with Trewe during her pregnancy, she experiences the strongest feelings of love she has ever known toward him, and she gazes repeatedly at the photograph of him that her husband later finds among her things. The reader knows the rational explanation for the subsequent resemblance of her child to Trewe (the adultery of which her husband suspects her) to be inaccurate; the correct explanation seems, instead, to rest in irrational connections between mind and body. Hardy's deployment of the specter of a maternal impression theory largely out of favor by the close of the nineteenth century positions women's mind and bodies as sites of unstable agency highly responsive to masculine force and easily misread under rubrics of rationalism.

Pregnancy and Syphilis in Victorian Literature, Culture, and Criticism

Although Victorian culture idealizes motherhood, pregnancy is largely hidden from view in mid-century novels. Pregnancy is also largely hidden from Victorian literary critical view, despite the field's deep investments in the analysis of gender, sexuality, and the body.[5] This narrative and critical elision attests to how effectively most Victorian texts work—as does Victorian maternity-wear—to conceal irrefutable physical evidence of female sexuality. Novels of the period tend to shield modest pregnant characters from the reader's gaze and only in instances of failure to conform to ideals of feminine modest and morality does the text retract some of its "protections."[6] Think, for example, of the revelation of willful Cathy Linton's pregnancy in Emily Brontë's (1847) *Wuthering Heights* or of the narration of Hetty Sorrel's premarital pregnancy in George Eliot's (1859) *Adam Bede*.

The legibility of Cathy and Hetty's pregnancies are exceptions to the general Victorian literary rule: the pregnancies of modest, white, middle-class characters are approached euphemistically if at all, as in the hesitant narration of Bella Wilfur's "ship upon the ocean" in Charles Dicken's (1865) *Our Mutual Friend* or the gentlest of hints (Sir James Chettam has "a little plan…to plead [his wife] Celia's indisposition as a reason for fetching Dorothea") that Celia is pregnant in Eliot's (1871) *Middlemarch*. The tendency toward euphemism is likely unsurprising to readers familiar with Victorian ideologies of class and gender and with literary reticence on matters sexual and somatic. Period narrations of illness are often exceptions that prove the rule of this reticence, treating embodied experience with detailed interest as a state more spiritual than fleshy. Indeed, where pregnancy is legible in the Victorian novel, it is often legible insofar as it maps onto illness and suffering, as in *Wuthering Heights* or in Elizabeth Gaskell's (1853) *Ruth*. Frank treatments of illness, however, do not extend to the depiction of syphilis. Like pregnancy, "the 'secret disease' was almost wholly excluded from [Victorian] literary works, and if it was alluded to, the author did so in an obscure manner, rarely describing bodily manifestations of the disease and never explicitly naming it" (Carpenter 2010, 72). "Never explicitly naming" conditions like pregnancy and syphilis that are widespread and impactful builds instability into the fabric of cultural ideology.

Jill L. Matus makes a case for the instability not only of representations of transgressive female sexuality and maternity—these representations tend to elide seemingly distinct categories of human and animal, "civilized" and "uncivilized," et cetera—but for the instability of these representations themselves. There is no "one way" in which dangerous sexuality and maternity is or can be represented. Matus sketches the connections between this instability in a seemingly ideologically coherent period and the broader shifts of modernity leading into a twentieth century in which ideological coherence proved increasingly elusive. Matus argues that the subversion of sexual ideology is baked into its very cultural creation:

> the [Victorian] notion of sexuality as culturally and environmentally responsive offered ways of defining differences among women of different classes, nationalities, and races. And given the instability of representations and their capacity to be used in oppositional or subversive contexts, ideas about unstable sexual difference were available to be mobilized to undermine the very ideologies with which they have been associated. (1995, 249)

Matus' close critical readings of bodies stop at George Eliot's *Middlemarch*, but her emphasis—as in the passage above—on the potential for the unstable representations of those bodies to "undermine" the stability of ideologies of gender, class, nation, and race gestures toward my investigation into the workings of pregnancy and syphilis in *The Heavenly Twins*.

At the *fin-de-siècle*, both pregnancy and syphilis became increasingly legible in literary narrative. The novels and stories of Olive Schreiner, George Egerton, Thomas Hardy, George Moore, George Gissing, and

Lucas Malet, for example, treat pregnancy as significant and fraught fodder for narrative. These narratives of pregnancy eschew earlier tendencies to position the condition as a gendered transgression of normative morality and focus, instead, on pregnant fears about the impressive, decadent power of the unconscious mind. Indeed, Clare Hanson ascribes the increasing legibility of syphilis in *fin-de-siècle* literature and culture to the period's anxieties about a decadent degeneracy (Hanson 2004, 83–85).

Though more narrative attention is granted to pregnancy and syphilis at the turn-of-the-century, that attention is seldom paid in somatic detail. As Andrew Smith notes, "Syphilis was a disease and a metaphor for disease…both a medical problem and a trope for social and cultural degeneration. In other words, there was the reality of the disease and a cultural fear of it" (2004, 95). The 1890s saw major shifts in normative ideologies, including the ideologies of gender, sexuality, bodies, and mind so central to shaping the ways pregnancy and sexuality are represented and the types of fears they evoke. These shifts changed the ways in which pregnancy and syphilis were depicted in novels of the period. Insofar as reading pregnancy and syphilis in *The Heavenly Twins* requires that we read immodesty and immorality, the locus of transgression has moved out of women's bodies and functions as the social disease of masculine transgression impressing itself upon the unspeakable spaces of women's minds and bodies. These forces shape pregnancy and syphilis on the canvas of women's minds and bodies, but those minds and bodies remain unknown in ways that signal a late-century shift toward concern with the dangers of the unconscious.

This shift reflects the emergence of and increasing cultural investment in the "New Psychology" that dates to the 1860s but converges markedly with medical practice, narrative form, and theories of gender and sexuality at the *fin-de-siècle*. As is the case, for example, in Freud's (1895) *Studies in Hysteria*, women's minds and bodies—often understood as such through their "ultimate" and "exceptional" ability to reproduce—serve the medical and emerging psychological field as backdrops against which to explore "the [blurred] line between body and mind," beyond the bodies and minds of women only (Mazzoni 2002, 24). Indeed, recent scholarship has explored the ways in which Victorians came, particularly at the close of the nineteenth century, to understand thinking in general as not necessarily conscious or brain-centric.[7]

Reading the intersection between *fin-de-siècle* pregnancy and syphilis in *The Heavenly Twins* gestures toward the ways in which the period expressed anxiety about impressions the unconscious might make on increasingly embattled expectations of "civilized" and "civilizing" progress. The 1890s saw an unraveling of popular faith in Imperial projects, in the gendered, middle-class mores and norms that had undergirded those projects, and the definitions of civilization upon which their rhetoric and practice relied. In this context, some of the strongest remaining arguments for the continued potential of progress may have rested on the huge strides in medical knowledge the nineteenth century had seen and that late-Victorians were beginning to perceive increasingly often in their daily lives and in the decreasing chances of premature death.[8] However, strides in medical knowledge were themselves increasingly tending toward an untethering of the knowable body of the patient from the knowing mind of the doctor and hinting at the perhaps unknowable powers of the unconscious minds of patients and doctors alike. As the Victorian period drew to a close, the anxieties evoked by textual representation of pregnancy and the societal prevalence of syphilis increasingly encompassed fears about the disruptive social and physical agency of the unconscious.

Though the Enlightenment had fostered a modern medical revolution and the creation of a new professional cadre of experts impressing their mental powers upon disorderly bodies, that discipline by the mid-/late-Victorian period had itself begun to verge increasingly upon a different order. Where mid-Victorian bodily symptoms were often understood as moral markers, late-Victorian bodies increasingly came to be understood by emerging psychological professionals and society at large as markers of disorderly minds and of larger social problems.[9] If the mind has the power to shape the body, then the cultivation of the mind might not lead only toward progress and improvement, but perhaps also toward degeneration and decadence that work according to an irrational calculus; futurity might not be shaped by the things we can see and say, but by the things we cannot.

That the unknowable space of pregnancy and syphilis is emphasized in the fiction of this period speaks both to a rising sense of, and also to a desire to control, the power over futurity wielded by the invisible and inarticulate. Pregnancy and syphilis in *The Heavenly Twins* also demonstrate the impossibilities of such control: one may see pregnant and syphilitic bodies and say what happens to them, and still not understand, much less control, their outcomes in any stable way.[10]

The Heavenly Twins

The Heavenly Twins is the didactic tale of a society that requires women's complete sexual innocence while encouraging male indiscretion. The ethereal Edith Beale is destroyed by her naïve parents' decision to allow her to marry the villainous Sir Mosely Menteith. Soon enervated by her marriage to a man who cannot contain his open interest in prostitutes even while walking with his young wife of less than a year, Edith's syphilitic decline first maddens, then kills her. Though Evadne Frayling survives the novel, her fine abilities are squandered when she is deceived about the character of her husband, Colonel Colquhoun. After learning of his moral turpitude on her wedding day, Evadne refuses to consummate her marriage and, over time, falls into a hysteria of sexual and mental repression. When Colquhoun dies suddenly, Evadne is able to enter into a seemingly satisfactory marriage with her doctor, Dr. Galbraith. She is not, however, able to regain the full measure of mental or physical health she enjoyed before her sacrifice on the altar of decadent male sexuality. Evadne's hysteria returns with a vengeance during her first pregnancy: she tries to kill herself and the unborn child she is convinced will be impressed by her exposure to "vice." Evadne's fears echo the fate of her friend, Edith. In *The Heavenly Twins,* syphilis works—through women's pregnant bodies and unconciouses—as a dangerous mechanism of impression upon futurity.

Syphilis in *The Heavenly Twins* "challenges gendered myths about the transmission of venereal disease, as well as dispelling female ignorance about this and other sexual matters" and makes legible a transition from mid-Victorian notions of stated pregnancy as a site of visible immorality toward *fin-de-siècle* notions of pregnancy as a site for the play of impression on vulnerable, permeable bodies (Hanson 2004, 88). In the novel, the immorality that circulates in women's reproductive bodies is not primarily their own but that of the society that is expected to protect them. As most critics have noted, *The Heavenly Twins* treats masculine immorality as an infectious social illness practically synonymous with syphilis.[11] In order to combat the spread of this disease through impressionable pregnant bodies, women must be able to see and say it; women must, in short, "read and diagnose the bodies of men 'exhausted by vice'" (269).

As Meegan Kennedy notes, however, Grand maintains the very reticence regarding explicit depictions of male syphilitic bodies which her novel decries. The infectious immorality that makes Edith and Evadne mentally and physically ill is primarily evidenced on both women's reproductive bodies. Edith's syphilitic decline is at first indistinguishable from a delayed post-partum recovery and Evadne's hysterical fears that there is "no past in the matter of vice, [that the] consequences become hereditary, and continue from generation to generation" surface most strongly during her first pregnancy, even though neither she nor Dr. Galbraith is personally guilty of sexual vice nor infected with syphilis (Grand 80). Although male sexual license is figured as a contagious disease, a degeneration that "moral…leper[s]" "help[] to spread" through the social body, the novel's narrative emphasizes the dangers posed to futurity through the impressions of that vice on women's pregnant bodies (2004, 79). One cannot read syphilis in Grand without reading pregnancy and the significance of the collaboration between the two is helpfully read through a lens of impression.

The Heavenly Twins figures the damage and degeneration caused by unread and unchecked syphilis in a language of bodily expansion:

> There are injuries which set up a carcinoma of the mind…cancer spots confined to a small area at first, but gradually extending with infinite pain until all the surrounding healthy tissue is more or less involved, and the whole beautiful fabric is absorbed in the morbid growth. (1992, 678)

This description of the "cancer" of the mind that results from the injury of contact with vice reads like the gothic narration of a pregnancy "gradually extending" into full-grown evil that consumes the "healthy tissue" of the mother. Such a "morbid growth," though referred to in the passage above with reference to Evadne's hysteria during her first pregnancy, also latches onto Edith after her marriage to Menteith and her post-partum decline. Edith's marriage takes place despite Evadne's strenuous objections to a man she felt to be legibly marked by vice. "I feel," Evadne argues with Edith and her mother, "I have some consciousness which informs me of things my intellect cannot grasp. And I do know [that he is bad—thoroughly bad]!" (232). Her inability to describe an uncanny sense of the evil Menteith will inevitably "set up" inside Edith speaks both to Grand's disinclination to represent the markers of syphilis on the bodies of men and also the impressive power of the illness and the male bodies that spread it on the minds and reproductive bodies of women.

Though Evadne can point to nothing concrete to which to object in the person of Menteith before his marriage to Edith, Edith's person is clearly—though indefinitely—marked by disease after it. A discussion between her parents names vague signs of syphilis on Edith's body only insofar as they name that body's post-partum condition:

> "That child [Edith] is not right," the Bishop said when Edith had gone to bed.
> "Have you noticed her face? I don't like the look of it at all; not at all."
> "Isn't that rather unkind, dear?" Mrs. Beale replied. "I always recovered in time."
> "You never were as ill as the poor child evidently is," he answered. (283)

Edith's face, which shows some definite sign of her syphilitic decline, is read by her parents as showing some indefinite sign of a failure to "recover" from childbirth in good "time." That the marks of illness are indeed definite is evidenced soon after when Angelica Hamilton-Wells—the novel's third heroine and the only one who, through denial of sexuality, fully escapes the dangers of syphilis—calls Edith "disfigured" (287). Though no one will speak the details of this disfigurement, of the something that is wrong with her face, there clearly *are* detailed, identifiable changes in Edith physical appearance.

That what those changes are, exactly, is never articulated directly, but rather gestured toward vaguely and repeatedly with increasing insistence echoes Edith's own knowing ignorance, a knowing ignorance the novel attacks as a mistakenly protected feminine state of mind. In speaking of her vague condition with her mother, Edith explains—in the longer section from which this chapter's epilogue is drawn—that diagnosis is intentionally withheld from her:

> "The doctor again!" Edith groaned. "It has been nothing but the doctor and 'tonics' ever since I have been married."
> "What does he say is the matter exactly?" Mrs. Beale asked.
> "All his endeavor seems to be not to say what is the matter exactly," Edith replied. (285)

The very reticence of the doctor to "say what is the matter exactly" speaks to its illicit nature. That "all his endeavor" must be put to the effort of concealing Edith's condition from Edith herself demonstrates that the doctor is not unaware of its cause but rather hyperaware. The doctor will not speak of syphilis to Edith because syphilis must not be spoken of to a lady, despite that lady's being in serious danger from it. In seeking to protect Edith's mind from the knowledge of syphilis, the doctor seeks to erect a barrier between mind and body than cannot hold, much as the narrative barrier between pregnant bodies and plot could not hold in mid-Victorian fiction: a pregnancy that skirts articulation nonetheless tends to result in the undeniable birth of a child. And Edith's case of syphilis, though it skirts direct articulation, nonetheless results in the undeniable degradation of two bodies.

The socio-medical ideal of a barrier between bodies and minds, particularly between privileged women's bodies and minds, maps onto matters of reproduction when Angelica's maidenly ignorance regarding babies emphasizes the unnameability of the problem with Edith's:

> Angelica had never been in the same house with a baby before, and she was all interest...
> 'Have you seen the baby?' she asked Elizabeth, when the latter was brushing her hair for dinner...
> 'Yes, Miss,' Elizabeth answered.
> 'Is he a pretty baby?' Angelica wanted to know.
> Elizabeth pursed her lips with an air of reserve.
> 'You don't think so?' Angelica said—she had seen the maid's face in the mirror before her.... (288)

Working-class Elizabeth clearly knows what Angelica does not, and—as a lady—ought not. As with the doctor whose reluctance to name "what is the matter exactly," Elizabeth's hesitance to speak of the baby's appearance suggests a specificity of her knowledge about its cause rather than a lack thereof. If she found him simply not a very pretty baby, there would be little cause for marked "reserve," a reserve expressed in the "purs[ing of] her lips" around something she knows but will not say. Angelica, "see[ing] the maid's face in the mirror," seems to understand that this reserve is weighted with significance. This understanding proves insufficient preparation for an encounter with the specific realities of the child's condition, however, much as Edith's education proved insufficient to prepare her for the reality of the social illness to which she unknowingly exposed herself in marrying Menteith. When Angelica does finally meet Edith's child, her "astonishment and horror" at the sight of a baby described as "old, old already and exhausted with suffering" drive her from the room, though they offer the reader a reference to a well-known symptom of syphilis in babies though without contextualizing that symptom explicitly or detailing the "suffering" with which it is associated (289).

The specific type of symptoms from which Edith's child is likely suffering are only ever spoken at a classed remove, through the description of an impoverished infant she sees at the side of the road with his equally ill and impoverished mother. This baby, "small and rickety, with bones that bent beneath its weight, slight as it was," is revealed by the dying mother to be the illegitimate son of Edith's husband. It is with this specific knowledge of male vice, knowledge from which her family and friends seek to protect her, that Edith is able to comprehend the nature of what is happening to her and her sick baby (290). Though she never names the syphilis that infects her and her child, Edith brings together the men in her life—her father, doctor, and husband—"who represent the arrangement of society which has made it possible for [her] and [her] child to be sacrificed in this way" in order to lay bare her knowledge of the disease they spread and allow to spread at their door (300).

The implied consummation of Edith's knowledge of syphilis does not, however, resolve all the elements of plot that are mysterious without this shared understanding of the unnamed workings of syphilis in the novel.

Though literary critics tend to speak of the disease as killing both Edith and her child over the course of the novel, there is actually an interesting lack of clarity about the fate of her baby. It is true that Evadne says of her disinclination to visit Edith's family home, Morningquest, that "Edith died there; and then that child" (590). This would make it seem that both Edith and the child are dead, or at least that Evadne thinks this is the case. However, not long after, Dr. Galbraith says that he "had seen how [Evadne] shrank from going to [Morningquest] because of the association with Edith's terrible death and the chance of seeing her poor, repulsive looking little boy there" (595). This would make it seem that the child is still living, but that Evadne has a strong aversion to seeing him. Perhaps her thinking him dead is a sign of the hysteria for which Galbraith is treating her by this point in the novel, a hysteria which comes to fixate on the dangers of syphilis to children. A later appearance of "Mrs. Beale… with Edith's boy" confirms either that the error is Evadne's—not a possibly careless Grand's—and/or that her "and then that child" might better be read, "and then that child…," the discontinued expression of a thought that it cuts itself off (677). This child seems, in fact, to be still alive at the novel's close, evidence of the threat posed to the future by social illness.

Unlike Edith, Evadne's marriage to a sexually impure man does not result in her contraction of syphilis. This may be due to her refusal to consummate her marriage to Colquohoun, a refusal based on the illicit medical education Evadne cobbled together for herself through adolescence, against the wishes of her parents. Though her body remains untainted by syphilis, however, Evadne's mind falls prey to a specter of the disease. In an echo of the prevalent syphilis "phobias" associated with the *fin-de-siècle*, Evadne fears that her "healthy tissue" has been irredeemably exposed to the carcinogen of Colquohoun's vice, a fear that peaks at a moment in which her own body, like that figurative cancer, is "gradually extending," "absorbed in the…growth" of generations (678).

Evadne's first pregnancy is explicitly exposed by her doctor-husband as salient evidence in his case study of her hysterical symptoms.[12] Unlike Edith, who remains unaware of her husband's moral cancer until shortly before her own death and whose pregnancy is skipped over entirely by the narrative in a formal demonstration of the danger that the unsaid and unseen poses to futurity, Evadne's pregnancy falls directly under the novel's narrative gaze. Dr. Galbraith's description of his treatment plan for Evadne emphasizes her physical body and hints at her condition, explaining that "there was active exercise enough for her…so long as she was able to take it, and when it became necessary to curtail the amount she drove both morning and afternoon, and took short walks." Dr. Galbraith also explains that he "began to hope that a new interest in life was coming to cure her of all morbid moods forever" (659). Of course, the new interest that Galbraith imagines will cure her and that curtails Evadne's active exercise is the child she carries. This kind of delicate revelation at the close of the century, though, evidences only a very gentle retraction of modest mid-Victorian textual conventions for the representation of pregnant bodies.

The full retraction of those conventions occurs only after Evadne attempts suicide, an act she is driven to after reading—against the advice of her doctor-husband—medical texts on the "heredity of vice" (662). I find Evadne's suicide attempt doubly suggestive: firstly, it is fueled by her desire to halt the heredity of vice she believes to be lodged and growing in her body after her exposure to her first husband's infectious immorality, an exposure that even her total chastity in her first marriage could not avoid, signaling her perception of the dangerous impressive powers of illness. Secondly, though this suicidal impulse is also framed by Dr. Galbraith as the result of male licentiousness, it is with a difference. Dr. Galbraith views the suicide attempt as a manifestation of the hysterical mental illness Evadne has contracted from her exposure to her first husband's vice, or rather, the hysteria that developed as a result of her desire to limit her sexual exposure to her husband's cancerous immorality. This is to say that the medical/psychological reading of the suicide attempt locates the very direct threat to futurity in Evadne's pregnant unconscious, pregnant both metaphorically (as containing depths hitherto hidden from husband and reader) and literally (as her unconscious while physically pregnant).

In any reading, Evadne's pregnant body is the site at which her own potential for moral illness, her exposure to an illness of the social body, and her resulting tendency toward mental illness is evidenced. After the vice that haunts her psyche is fully revealed, so too is her pregnant body fully exposed to the medical gaze of her husband, the psychological specialist Sir Shadwell Rock, and the reader. Her pregnancy makes the sinister hold of syphilis on her mind legible, and the sinister hold of syphilis on her mind makes the embodied details of her pregnancy legible. This collaboration is psychologically and narratively motived by the threat that illness will impress itself upon the body of Evadne's unborn child. Of course, this threat is real enough, though likely not in the way Evadne imagines. The mental illness Evadne experiences in reaction to the dangers and damages of syphilis in her world leads her to attempt to destroy both herself and her unborn child. At the novel's conclusion, Evadne—though the somewhat stabilized mother of two—has not been able to fully resolve this threat for herself; the unwritten future remains endangered by a disease that cannot be wholly known or articulated, a disease that Evadne imagines circulating in her body but that her husband locates in her mind.

For the "forty-six days and nights" that remain of Evadne's first pregnancy, however, Dr. Galbraith explains with chronological precision uncharacteristic in earlier Victorian narrations of reproduction, "[he] never left her an hour alone" (666). Dr. Galbraith's constant supervision of Evadne during the final six weeks of her pregnancy is made possible by their marital relationship—even the most dedicated doctor would not be able to commit six weeks of constant care to only one patient—but that constant supervision is motivated by a complicated mix of his function as husband, as a father-to-be, as doctor, and as nascent psychologist. These mixed motivations signal the slippage between Dr. Galbraith's role as medical professional and as upper-middle-class domestic partner. Evadne herself has already remarked upon this fuzzy distinction, declaring that "it is so anomalous being both a doctor and a country gentleman" (569). Indeed, the courtship of Evadne and Dr. Galbraith is conducted on the slippery surface of his shifting professional and private roles, complicated by the conflicting codes of modesty that govern a woman's relationship with her doctor and a woman's relationship with any other man. "A doctor is not a man to his lady patients," Evadne declares, "but an abstraction—a kindly abstraction for whom one sends when a man's presence would be altogether inconvenient" (570). Clearly, a doctor may see and know things that a *man* may not and can be depended upon "not to say what the matter is exactly" when to do so would be inappropriate. Indeed, in an instance when Dr. Galbraith calls upon Evadne socially, she excoriates her "stupid" maid for having thought that he was coming to see her professionally and ushering him into her bedroom (577). Evadne's attempts to relegate Dr. Galbraith's diagnostic gaze on her body to his professional function and away from their personal relationship are as unsuccessful once they are married as they were before. Indeed, Dr. Galbraith's medical function in the novel slips smoothly into his function as Evadne's husband and narrator, though his success in all three roles is tenuous.

Our "success" in reading Evadne's pregnant body here is tenuous, too. Certain physical and chronological information is more readily available than it was in mid-Victorian fiction, but that doesn't seem to help us read the pregnancy's somatic particularities, just as the novel's descriptions of syphilis don't much help us to read the specific symptoms of the illness. Both syphilis and pregnancy function primarily, rather, as metaphorical conditions of minds and dangerously permeable social bodies. The true source of threat to a pregnant Evadne and her unborn child—her unconscious, the impressions of a degenerate society upon that unconscious, and the power the unconscious holds over life and death—remains largely illegible due to its insistence on a permeability of body and mind that post-Enlightenment logic resists. Our diagnosis of Evadne's pregnancy—as her own diagnosis of her infection with vice—is only ever partial and tends toward its own metaphoricization. This is a pattern of metaphoricization with which the reader of *The Heavenly Twins* is already familiar, having been carefully instructed throughout the novel's pages in the reading of syphilis as a marker for diseased society. Much as Evadne imagines Edith's child dead before his time, we must imagine syphilis as alive (in Evadne) where it is not if we are to make sense of her hysteria; we do this through thinking its impressive power on the futurity promised and threatened by her pregnant body.

Notes

1. William Driscoll connects syphilis as metaphor with women's reproductive bodies: As a result the medical community, despite extensive scientific evidence to the contrary, repeatedly portrayed female reproductive

organs as the site of contamination, a portrayal that reinforced, both in law and social taboos, the double standard that simultaneously allowed male profligacy while enforcing feminine virtue (2009).

2. Mazzoni also employs this passage from Oakley.
3. Though Marie-Helene Huet traces maternal impression theories from the classical age though the modern one, Mazzoni cautions that such a lineage conflates maternal impression with a "different, ancient theory" that what a couple or woman saw during conception marked the fetus (1993, 16).
4. Wilson writes about the influence of notions of maternal impression on Fielding, Sterne, and Smollett: the maternally derived birthmark in Fielding's *Joseph Andrews* ultimately reveals the true identity of a main character. Jonathan Wild, Fielding's protagonist in his 1745 novel of the same name, has his whole criminal future impressed upon him by his mother's "violent desires to acquire all sorts of property" during her pregnancy. Sterne's novel, *Tristam Shandy*, also concerns an individual whose life is marked via in utero influence, a point that readers learn from the opening pages of the work. Tobias Smollett, a trained surgeon and physician, presents a more elaborate account of the action of maternal impression upon the character development of his protagonist, Peregrine Pickle. Smollett's attention to maternal matters in this work is understandable given that, while composing *Peregrine Pickle*, he was concurrently editing and annotating a Treatise on the Theory and Practice of Midwifery for the Edinburgh physician and male midwife, William Smellie, to whom he had served as an apprentice (Wilson 2002, 10).
5. Two notable exceptions to the lack of scholarly work on Victorian representations of pregnancy are Clare Hanson's (2004) *A Cultural History of Pregnancy: Pregnancy Medicine and Culture (1750–2000)* and Cynthia Northcutt Malone's (2000) "Near Confinement: Pregnant Women in the Nineteenth-Century British Novel" both of which treat the general tendency of Victorian novels to elide the representation of pregnancy to associate it with immorality.
6. This is an argument I make at more length in my dissertation, "Heavy Expectations: Reading Pregnancy in the Victorian Novel" and in "Now You See It: Concealing and Revealing Pregnancy in *Wuthering Heights* and the *Clever Woman of the Family*" (2015).
7. The revelation that Vanessa Ryan plagiarized sections of her influential *Thinking Without Thinking in the Victorian Novel* troubles the

debt this chapter owes to her work on what she calls the "not wholly agential or wholly conscious" thinking that occurs in Victorian fiction, thinking Ryan's book demonstrates "is not confined solely to the brain" (2012, 13). That the plagiarism in the book seems to have been in sections dealing with the details of Victorian scientific thinking supports Ryan's claims, I think, that the argumentative thrust of her book is legitimate—this argumentative thrust is certainly one with which this chapter is in conversation. This is a conversation, however, that need hardly rely wholly upon Ryan's work as Elisha Cohn's forthcoming *Still Life: Suspended Development in the Victorian Novel* and Anne McCarthy's work on suspension in nineteenth-century poetry attest.

8. See Mary Wilson Carpenter's *Health, Medicine, and Society in Victorian England* for more on these shifts.
9. For an example of prevalent Victorian assumptions regarding the relationship between "medicine and morality," Matus points to Elizabeth Blackwell's 1884 assertion that "medicine and morality being relation to function and use, are therefore inseparable in a Christian State" (2009, 2).
10. This vocabulary of "see" and "say" is drawn, as is much of the scholarship with which this chapter engages, from Michel Foucault's *Birth of the Clinic* in which he treats shifts in ways of seeing and saying that follow the codification of medical education in the eighteenth century. Foucault argues that "a new alliance was forged between words and things, enabling one *to see* and *to say*" (1994, xii; emphasis Foucault's). The ability of a specialized few to see and to say enabled, in turn says Foucault, the development of a medical gaze that codified separations of mind and body.
11. In addition to the work of Meegan Kennedy, William Driscoll, and Clare Hanson I draw upon here, see also, for example, Emma Liggins "Writing against the 'husband-fiend': syphilis and male sexual vice in the new woman novel" and Carol A. Senf's "Introduction" to the 1992 edition of *The Heavenly Twins*.
12. Malone (2000) has noted that the reticent narration of Celia's pregnancy in *Middlemarch* in contrast with the more direct narration of Rosamond's can be ascribed to the "narrative zone of the doctor-husband"; I draw here on this terminology.

References

Blackwell, Elizabeth. 1894. *Human Element in Sex: Being a Medical Inquiry Into the Relation of Sexual Physiology to Christian Morality*. London: Churchill.

Carpenter, Mary Wilson. 2010. *Health, Medicine, and Society in Victorian England*. Santa Barbara: Praeger.

Cohn, Elisha. 2012. Still Life: Suspended Animation in Charlotte Brontë's Villette. *SEL Studies in English Literature 1500–1900* 52 (4): 843–860.

Driscoll, William. 2009. The Metaphor of Syphilis in Grand's Heavenly Twins. *Nineteenth-Century Gender Studies* 5 (1): n. pag.

Eliot, George. (1871) 2000. *Middlemarch*, ed. Bert G. Hornbach. New York/ London: W.W. Norton.

Foucault, Michel. (1963) 1994. *The Birth of the Clinic: An Archaeology of Medical Perception*. New York: Vintage Books, 1994.

Freud, Sigmund, Josef Breuer, and Rachel Bowlby. 2004. *Studies in Hysteria*. Trans. Nicola Luckhurst. 1st Printing edition. London/New York: Penguin Classics.

Grand, Sarah. (1893) 1992. *The Heavenly Twins*. Ann Arbor: University of Michigan Press.

Hanson, Clare. 2004. *A Cultural History of Pregnancy: Pregnancy, Medicine, and Culture, 1750–2000*. New York: Palgrave Macmillan.

Hardy, Thomas. 1894. An Imaginative Woman. *The Pall Mall Magazine*: 951–969.

Huet, Marie Hélène. 1993. *Monstrous Imagination*. Cambridge: Harvard University Press.

Kennedy, Meegan. 2010. *Revising the Clinic: Vision and Representation in Victorian Medical Narrative and the Novel*. Columbus: Ohio State University Press.

Liggins, Emma. 2000. Writing against the 'husband-Fiend': Syphilis and Male Sexual Vice in the New Woman Novel. *Women's Writing* 7 (2): 175–195.

Malone, Cynthia Northcutt. 2000. Near Confinement: Pregnant Women in the Nineteenth-Century British Novel. *Dickens Studies Annual* 29: 367–385.

Matus, Jill L. 1995. *Unstable Bodies: Victorian Representations of Sexuality and Maternity*. New York: St. Martin's Press.

Mazzoni, Cristina. 2002. *Maternal Impressions: Pregnancy and Childbirth in Literature and Theory*. Ithaca: Cornell University Press.

Oakley, Ann. 1985. *The Captured Womb: History of the Medical Care of Pregnant Women*. New York: Blackwell Publishers.

Ryan, Vanessa L. 2012. *Thinking without Thinking in the Victorian Novel.* Baltimore: Johns Hopkins University Press.

Senf, Carol A. 1992. Introduction. In *The Heavenly Twins*. Ann Arbor: University of Michigan Press.

Smith, Andrew. 2004. *Victorian Demons: Medicine, Masculinity, and the Gothic at the* Fin-de-Siècle, 1st edn. Manchester: Manchester University Press.

Wilson, Philip K. 2002. (Philip Kevin). Eighteenth-Century 'Monsters' and Nineteenth-Century 'Freaks': Reading the Maternally Marked Child. *Literature and Medicine* 21 (1): 1–25.

Woods, Livia Arndal. 2015. Now You See It: Concealing and Revealing Pregnancy in Wuthering Heights and The Clever Woman of the Family. *Victorian Network* 6 (1 Summer): 32–54.

Unspeakable Horror: Outing Syphilis in Joseph Conrad's *Heart of Darkness*

Nicole Cosentino and Wendy Ryden

Heart of Darkness (1902) is a novella suffused with imagery of death. From the unnamed and fictionalized Brussels dubbed the "sepulchral city," to the rotting corpses littering the African landscape, to the depiction of the Intended being swallowed up in the encroaching darkness of the dead Kurtz's unspoken words, death haunts the narrative. As with most aspects of the novel, critics tend to interpret such gothic imagery metaphysically, arguing, for example, that Conrad "employing death as a metaphor for disillusionment, or spiritual extinction, . . . chronicles the failure of human intentions and lofty aspirations" (Billy 1997, 71). But if, as Ted Billy argues, Kurtz's horror "has as many meanings as interpreters" (1997, 73), perhaps it is time to attend to the possibility that Conrad's

N. Cosentino (✉)
University at Albany, Albany, NY, USA

W. Ryden
Long Island University Post, Brookville, NY, USA

K. Nixon, L. Servitje (eds.), *Syphilis and Subjectivity*,
https://doi.org/10.1007/978-3-319-66367-8_7

vision of death in this work includes a literal one, too, besides and intertwined with the obvious colonial violence being perpetrated in and on the Congo. In this view, Europe is not dying just of a vaguely defined spiritual anemia or moral corruption but of a physical illness that is equally perceived as threatening the ideals of civilization. While the horror exposed through Marlow's journey may very well be the indeterminacy of experience and relativity of truth, the evil within, or the existential hollowness of modernity, it may simultaneously refer to something all too tangible, pervasive, and identifiable: syphilis, the disease that the late Victorian population understood as a degenerative menace to Western civilization itself.

> The state of knowledge concerning syphilis in the final decades of the [nineteenth] century . . . was conducive to pessimism, if not medical nihilism. In the mid nineteenth century, the leading European authority. Philippe Ricord, an eminent French syphilologist, had promoted a basically optimistic model of syphilis as limited, treatable and controllable. However, his successor, Alfred Fournier, presented an altogether more pervasive and pessimistic view. . . .Syphilis therefore came to operate as a potent cultural metaphor for complex feelings of *fin de siècle* unease on an international scale. (Davidson and Hall 2001, 5)

Thus while "the horror of genocide and torture in King Leopold's Congo" certainly constitutes, to say the least, a significant "historical reality . . . behind Marlow's narrative" (Greaney 2002, 73), so too is the Victorian fear of syphilis and the silence surrounding it a potent historical exigency to consider in our readings of this work, especially as it dovetails with Conrad's motifs of primitivism and ineffability.

Bernard J. Paris poses the question, "What is it that is driving Marlow?" (2005, 17), and after rejecting several possibilities, concludes that it is the darkness itself that attracts the young captain, that is to say the danger, which is "deadly," according to Paris, and that Marlow welcomes the chance "to show that he is man enough to face the darkness" (2005, 18). If we accept that syphilis as well as other life-threatening sexually transmitted diseases set up a necrophiliac dynamic between danger and sex, then Paris's seemingly innocent pronouncement about Marlow's manhood takes on a particular cast, one in which erotic implications are restored to the notion of testing masculinity in the space of the eroticized Primitive, a colonial space, as Edward Said suggested of the Orient, that holds the possibility of "free" sex, perceived as unencumbered by Europe's regulatory bourgeois apparatus (1979, 190). Thus, the darkness that Marlow and Kurtz face is the darkness of desire and the Victorian understanding of desire's deadly consequences. Marlow witnesses first-hand the results of Kurtz's indulgence: the descent into madness and the indignity of his forsaken death, a disease progression that parallels what would have been recognized in the nineteenth century as tertiary syphilis—the disease that Deborah Hayden has referred to as the era's "dark secret" (2004, xv) and what Charles Crow calls "the unmentionable disease that haunted the Victorian period" on both sides of the Atlantic (2009, 110).

While knowledge of tropical diseases such as malaria and dysentery, not to mention the reputed effects of "the climate" in general, certainly influenced Conrad's and other Europeans' idea of jungle contagions, the fear of disease manifested in the novella need not be limited to these sources. After all, despite its association with sexual activity, syphilis, at the turn of century, remained something of a mystery:

> While bacteriologists were identifying the causative organisms of many illnesses, the origin of syphilis remained unknown. As many of the case studies document, throughout Europe the persistence of syphilis (like that of tuberculosis and cancer) fed into the anxieties fueled by Darwinian doctrines. If the concept of survival of the fittest initially seemed to confer an evolutionary basis for the superiority of the industrialized West, it also posed the threat that other organisms might endanger that hegemony. Thus eugenic and degenerationist discourses at the turn of the century were powerfully influenced by the increasing apparent congenital ravages of syphilis. (Davidson and Hall 2001, 6)

Perhaps it hardly needs to be said, but as John Stape argues, although models have been proposed for Kurtz, the character "was assembled from the scattered bits and pieces of things observed, read and imagined," and the story is "not a documentary account of selected events witnessed by Conrad, and still less a work of social realism" (2007, 66). Just as Conrad's work exceeds the limitations of a travel narrative to become an allegory for the evils of its time, so too may the portrayal of "jungle fever" be expansive to include projections about the contagion that represented fears of physical and moral degeneracy, important themes in Conrad's work. Such a reading becomes particularly compelling when we consider that Conrad overtly eroticized his narrative by including the detail of the native "mistress," or "Amazon" as Chinua Achebe has referred to her, as being integral to Kurtz's downfall, a detail underscored by the counterpoint of the chaste Intended vainly awaiting his return. It was, in other words, not merely "the climate" that produced Kurtz's tragedy nor was he seduced merely by the temptations of a white man given unfettered power to acquire ivory. Libidinal energy runs deep through Conrad's tale of "no restraint."

Conrad's deployment in his text of a sole African woman to signify the dangerously erotic is consistent with nineteenth-century European views of African sexuality as "primitive, uncontrolled and excessive," and representative of "the darkness and dangers of the continent."[1] Critics have argued that the figure of the black woman evoked for white Europeans the fear of rampant sexuality and the post-Darwinian preoccupation with degeneracy into a primitive state (Vaughan 1991, 129–130). In his report describing the syphilis epidemic that was afflicting the Bagandan people in the early twentieth century, F.J. Lambkin, a colonel in the British Royal Army Medical Corps, blamed the prevalence of the disease on colonial intrusion into traditional tribal hierarchy that unleashed the sexuality of black women, who "were merely female animals with strong passions" now given "unrestricted opportunities" for gratification (qtd. in Vaughan 1991, 133). Seen in this light, Conrad's African mistress functions as yet another problematic aspect of his colonial critique: the European presence in the dark continent has liberated from tribal hierarchy dangerous black female sexuality to prey upon white European men, as seen in this description:

> She walked with measured steps, draped in striped and fringed cloths, treading the earth proudly, with a slight jingle and flash of barbarous ornaments… She was savage and superb, wild-eyed and magnificent… And in the hush that had fallen suddenly upon the whole sorrowful land… the

colossal body of the fecund and mysterious life seemed to look at her, pensive, as though it had been looking at the image of its own tenebrous and passionate soul. (Conrad 2008, 101–02)

The erotic thread that runs through *Heart of Darkness* is not limited to heterosexual expression. We can trace as well the homosocial/erotic desire manifested by Marlow toward Kurtz and through other characters. Marlow's impulse to "find" Kurtz becomes, after all, one of the primary devices that Conrad uses to propel the plot. As Andrew Michael Roberts says, "the focus of horror is . . . Marlow's intense emotional desire to meet Kurtz" (133). Following Nina Pelikan Straus's lead in reading Marlow's desire for Kurtz as part of the dark unspeakable horror of the novella, Roberts states frankly that "an interpretation of 'Heart of Darkness' in terms of male homosexual desire can undoubtedly be made," and that the work is filled with "distinctly sexual overtones within the discourse of sexuality/knowledge that [Eve Kosofsky] Sedgwick identifies in late nineteenth-century Europe" (131). Thus, Marlow is a seaman whose thrill of exploration culminates in his quest for the colonial prodigy, Kurtz. Throughout Marlow's voyage, we, as readers, see a gradual buildup of Marlow's sexual determination to retrieve Kurtz and then witness that same determination become negated by Kurtz's deterioration and obvious union with the African mistress and implied relationship with the Russian harlequin. This negation, one of many "horrors" that present themselves throughout the novella, extinguishes Marlow's fantasies about an erotic union with Kurtz. To Marlow, Kurtz is now a shadow of a man, a man who had voluntarily (and more than likely, jubilantly) had sex with women and men for pleasure and power. If Kurtz represents the degenerate, overly sexualized immoral figure, Marlow is virtually no better in his hypocritical valorization of hegemonic norms that are paradoxically sexualized in his admiration for and pursuit of Kurtz. That Marlow is placed in the role of the hypocrite is important, given his professed disdain for this aspect of civilization that constitutes part of the basis for his obsession with the unapologetic Kurtz.

Through Marlow's voyage of self-discovery, we can see the sexual tension among Conrad's male characters, including the African "backdrop" characters who are noted for their muscular physicality. Vivid diction surrounding male-on-male encounters is indicative of masked and displaced homosexual desire. We learn that Marlow was "rather excited at the prospect of meeting Kurtz very soon" (54) even as his anxiety is revealed in his frustration over the impotence of his ship, "the wretched thing" which he "expected . . . to give up every moment" (62). Marlow alludes to the Russian harlequin's relationship with Kurtz as being an intimate one; he recalls the Russian telling him of the private moments that he and Kurtz had shared prior to Marlow's arrival. As a result, Marlow finds himself "seduced into something like admiration—like envy" (91). Almost as though verging on a kind of awareness of homosocial desires, Marlow retreats from his aforementioned statements in an effort to seek validation and justification for the possible misinterpretation of his words: "I did not envy him his devotion to Kurtz… I must say that to me it appeared about the most dangerous thing in every way he had come upon so far" (92).

This tango between jealousy and denial continues throughout the quest for Kurtz. Similarly, the harlequin revokes his statement that he and Kurtz spoke of love by saying to Marlow, "It's not what you think" and replaces the idea with the vagary: "he made me see things—things" (92).[2] The harlequin's description of Kurtz reads like that of mercurial, abusive lover: "sometimes he would take to me; sometimes it was better for me to be careful" (94), and he describes, as though it were a harem squabble, the competition that exists between him and his "erotic rival" (Ruppel 2008, 32), the African mistress, for Kurtz's favor: "I have been risking my life everyday for a fortnight to keep her out of the house. . . . she talked like a fury to Kurtz for an hour, pointing at me" (2008, 103).[3] Yet Marlow's sexuality, unlike the Russian harlequin's and the mistress's, remains liminal and closeted in the cloaked guise of Victorian gender norms despite the uncanny intrusion of his emotional response. When Marlow believes he might miss out on meeting Kurtz at all, he tells us "my sorrow had a startling extravagance" and that "I couldn't have felt more of lonely desolation had I been robbed of a belief or had missed my destiny in life" (78). But in the end, Marlow's "active refusal to identify with his sexual other" pushes him toward alignment with a "safer homosocial network with inbuilt racist and postcolonial ideals" (Mitchell and O'Rourke 2011, 84).

As Marlow and the harlequin become better acquainted, Marlow asserts that the intercourse between the harlequin and Kurtz "had been very much broken by various causes," and Marlow seems annoyed that the harlequin "managed to nurse Kurtz through two illnesses" (93). Marlow's ambivalence toward the apparent relationship between the Russian and Kurtz is revealed in his deprecating comparison of them to two ships that had "come together unavoidably" and "lay rubbing sides" (92). This relationship essentially serves as Kurtz's outing. We learn that

> the wilderness had found him out early, and had taken on him a terrible vengeance for the fantastic invasion. I think it had whispered to him things about himself which he did not know, things of which he had no conception till he took counsel with this great solitude—and the whisper had proved irresistibly fascinating. (96–97)

Kurtz is glorified throughout the novella in a hyper masculine, domineering manner, which makes him seem god-like and nearly intangible. But through Marlow's jealousy, we are exposed to the problematized bisexuality of Kurtz as well as Marlow's own uncertainty about his attraction to Kurtz. Marlow repeatedly expresses his fascination with Kurtz in terms of confused, secret desire and defilement as when he attempts to retrieve the escaped Kurtz: "—and to this day I don't know why I was so jealous of sharing with anyone the peculiar blackness of that experience" (108). His confusion continues when he ponders what he planned to do upon actually uniting with Kurtz, offering an acceptable, masculinist explanation that he would give "him a drubbing," although Marlow's embarrassment at the inadequacy of this cover story seems almost palpable: "I don't know. I had some imbecile thoughts" (108). In fact, this incident lays "the foundations of . . . [their] intimacy . . . to endure" (110).

It becomes clear, then, that *Heart of Darkness* is a haunted work, riddled with gothic anxiety about desire and the forbidden. If it is an eroticized narrative, it is equally a necrotized one, in which desire and death appear inextricable, a point driven home by Cedric Watts's comparison of the vampire imagery in "The Heart of Darkness,"[4] in which Kurtz is portrayed as the "undead" (2012, 9) to that found in Bram Stoker's *Dracula*. For example, this image of the demented, dying Kurtz (whom Marlow refers to earlier as being "disinterred" [Conrad 2008, 79]), while perversely evocative of Christ in the tomb, also suggests demonic resurrection.[5]

> His covering had fallen off, and his body emerged from it pitiful and appalling as from a winding-sheet. I could see the cage of his ribs all astir, the bones of his arm waving. It was as though an animated image of death carved out of old ivory had been shaking its hand with menaces at a motionless crowd of men made of dark and glittering bronze. I saw him open his mouth wide—it gave him a weirdly voracious aspect, as though he had wanted to swallow all the air, all the earth, all the men before him. (Conrad 2008, 99–100)

As Sara Wasson points out, "vampiric contagion" has long been understood as a Victorian projection "of the anxieties concerning sexual infection, particularly. . . syphilis" (2014, 135). Watt's identification here of Stoker's influence on Conrad further suggests that fear of syphilis informs Conrad's vision of the horror that haunts the civilized world, for just as in the case of *Dracula*, fear of disease contagion mingles in colonial discourse with fear of the exoticized other. It is important to stress here that we are not arguing for a reading of *Heart of Darkness* as a syphilis narrative on a literal level, for certainly a real-life counterpart to Kurtz could not have contracted and progressed through the disease in the short period that he remained in Africa, although it is possible to speculate that he might have contracted it long before leaving Europe while he was still the renowned progressive idealist. Such hypocrisy would certainly be within the thematic scope of Conrad's work. But our reading is not based on this speculation. Rather we are asserting that the symptoms Kurtz exhibits and Marlow's response to them are consistent with manifestations of and reactions to a pervasive disease shrouded in silence and shame, a disease that Conrad would have certainly been aware of but would not have spoken about overtly, a disease connected with fears of degeneracy and the perils of colonialism and exploration, and as such might be a likely model for Conrad to draw upon in creating his portrait of Kurtz's allegorical affliction.

Although Conrad's letters and journals reveal a concern over his own health, especially in relation to travel, he makes no mention of syphilis, nor would we expect him to. According to Deborah Hayden, despite the prevalence of the disease in Europe, "The word was taboo, with the terrifying diagnosis at most whispered to an intimate friend, and then only with assurances of utmost secrecy. It was too shameful to record by name in a diary and was alluded to in correspondence only in code" (2004, xv). There is of course nothing to suggest that Conrad himself was concerned about having the disease, but he must certainly have been aware of the threat it posed and the stigma attached to it. As Stape points out, Maupassant, in the last stages of syphilis, arrived for treatment at Champelles-les bains outside of Geneva shortly after Conrad finished his own recuperative stint there in 1891 (2007, 68). While their visits did not overlap, Conrad must have understood that guests were being treated for such afflictions. Interestingly, around this time, Conrad had taken up residence in what he himself saw as a seamy part of London in proximity of brothels, an area he described as "hot, noisy and dissipated" (Stape 2007, 68). Given the negative reception in England of a work like Ibsen's *Ghosts*, which directly takes on the syphilitic plot and was condemned as immoral for its troubles, it is unlikely Conrad would attempt such a risk even if he was consciously aware of a desire to do so.

The silence surrounding syphilis is attested to in numerous sources and illustrated graphically in the anonymous memoir, *My Secret Life*, an example of Victorian erotica that is heralded as an important cultural document for its graphic detail that allows us to glimpse the underside of this silenced topic. Written sometime in the last decades of the century, it was first published around the turn of the century. The author piles up detail after detail in a meticulous description of a prodigious sexual life starting from youth. The author establishes very early some enduring Victorian motifs: a fascination with filth and sexuality and violence, and an overwhelming fear of disease and degeneracy. In the first chapters, the author tells us of the fear of sexually transmitted and associative disease being driven into him by his godfather and others, and the accompanying fear of discovery attesting to the imperative to keep secret this great malady: "the pox." The narrator "Walter" writes to his cousin Fred of his anxiety over discovering the joys of masturbation. Fred replies that "some fellows at his school had been caught at it, and flogged; that a big boy just going to Oxford had had a woman and got the pox badly. He begged me to burn his letter, or throw it down the shithouse directly I had read it" (*My Secret Life* ch 4). After Walter's first sexual encounter in which he rapes a maid named Charlotte, his success is marred by the thought of infection: "I took it into my head, that Charlotte had given me some disease, and was in a dreadful state of mind" (ch 5). The memoir reflects both the prevalence of the disease as well the shame and guilt associated with it.

While *Heart of Darkness* never specifies what affliction has befallen Kurtz, the many references in the text to "the climate," something Conrad himself was very concerned with, suggest that he has succumbed to some sort of jungle fever that has contributed to his "going native." The melding of the notion of jungle fever and syphilitic infection is present from the very beginnings of the colonial enterprise in the story of Columbus himself and his perils in the New World. Whether European syphilis was a direct consequence of Columbus's voyages remains undetermined, but the idea of Columbus and his crew as progenitors of the disease on the Continent was advanced in Europe as early as the eighteenth century (Arrizabalaga et al. 1997, 11), given that "the drama and horror of the syphilis epidemic in Europe began soon after Columbus and his crew sailed into the harbor of Palos, Spain, on 15 March 1493" (Hayden 2004, 5). In her conjecture about whether Columbus suffered from syphilis, Deborah Hayden notes that he became afflicted with an ongoing illness that coincided with his despotic treatment of the inhabitants of Hispaniola, which she describes as a "reign of terror with beheadings and burnings at the stake. Bodies hung from gallows in every town on Hispaniola" (2004, 7).

This description of Columbus's ruthlessness matches Kurtz's cruelty and recklessness in Conrad's novella with perhaps an added twist: Marlow describes the impalement of human heads on spikes turned not outward[6] as a traditional inducement of fear and warning but rather inward for the sake of Kurtz's own perverse pleasure, a further sign of inward retreat that we might associate with the dementia of tertiary syphilis. While there is no shortage of historical despotic personalities for Conrad to draw on for inspiration, it seems that Conrad might find Columbus a compelling figure, and indeed his tyranny in Hispaniola echoes Kurtz's reign in the Congo as described by Conrad. As interested as he was in exploration, Conrad perhaps knew something of Columbus's voyages.[7] In his essay "Geography and Some Explorers," Conrad presents this ambiguous view:

> The greatest of them all, who has presented modern geography with a new world to work upon, was at one time loaded with chains and thrown into prison. Columbus remains a pathetic figure, not a sufferer in the cause of geography, but a victim of the imperfections of jealous human hearts, accepting his fate with resignation. Among explorers he appears lofty in his troubles and like a man of a kingly nature. His contribution to the knowledge of the earth was certainly royal. . . . [even] if the discovery of America was the occasion of the greatest outburst of reckless cruelty and greed known to history. (1926, 4)

It is clear from this passage that while Conrad was acutely aware of and deplored the devastation wrought by the colonization of the New World, he also admired Columbus's feat in facing what in the African conquest is called "the darkness." Columbus, like Kurtz, is not guilty of falling prey to "a flabby, pretending, weak-eyed devil of a rapacious and pitiless folly" but rather exhibits the robust evil—"the devil of violence, and the devil of greed, and the devil of hot desire . . . strong, lusty, red-eyed devils, that swayed and drove men—men, I tell you" (2008, 24)—that Marlow begrudgingly respects in comparison to, to use Hannah Arendt's phrase *avant la lettre*, the banality of evil exhibited by the Station Manager and other hypocritical bureaucrats in the Company.

Conrad's attitude here toward Columbus is not unlike Marlow's toward Kurtz: an envy and admiration mixed with abhorrence and disgust. Likewise, just as Conrad sees envy as contributing to Columbus's fate, Kurtz too is a victim of "jealous human hearts." This point is made particularly clear in the novella when Marlow learns through his eavesdropping that the Station Manager and his uncle have engaged in covert sabotage of Kurtz in order to eliminate him as competition.[8] Thus we see marked similarities between Columbus and Kurtz and Conrad's and Marlow's attitudes toward each, respectively: the cruel, bizarre behavior that culminates in the tragic, ignominious decline of the favored, and then finally discredited, trailblazer, a trajectory, in the case of Columbus and, we believe in the case of Kurtz, too, that is explainable by and perceived to be a result of syphilitic infection.

In the abandonment of conventional moral standards, Columbus, like Kurtz, bears pronounced resemblance to the figure of Friedrich Nietzsche's *ubermensch*, and this points us to another possible source for the inspiration behind Kurtz and, as it happens, another suspected syphilitic. The influence of Nietzsche on Conrad has long been accepted: "That Conrad knew of Nietzsche has never been in doubt; between 1899 and 1919 Conrad refers to him in several letters and one published essay" (Butte 1989, 161). The particular influence on *Heart of Darkness*, especially with regard to Kurtz and the *ubermensch* or superman concept, has been definitively articulated by George B. Alexander in his indisputable demonstration of the appearance of Nietzschean phrases and ideas, such as the "whited sepulcher" (1980, 105), that would have been available to Conrad, if not directly through Nietzsche's work, then through secondary publications that Conrad would have been familiar with: "Nietzsche would have been inescapable for a reader like Conrad, who not only read widely but also picked up what was current in intellectual circles at the time. Around the turn of the century Nietzsche was widely known throughout Europe" (Renner 2012, 146). That Conrad was dismissive of Nietzsche is also true as he disparagingly declared in his 1901 letter to Ford Maddox [Heuffer] Ford, "That's what Niet[z]sche's phil [osophy] leads to—here's your overman" (1986, vol. 2, 344) and in an 1899 letter, he references "The mad individualism of Niet[z]sche" (188). George Butte concludes, "Conrad's relation to Nietzsche is then a mixed and unstable one; it includes attraction and suspicion, revision and distortion" (1989, 168), not unlike, as we have seen, Marlow's response to Kurtz.

The similarities between Kurtz and the *ubermensch* are legion and obvious as Kurtz epitomizes the man positioned beyond the judgment of a Christian morality that has masked the true Darwinian nature of the world where the will to power triumphs and the weak are eliminated or dominated. Conrad's rendering of the primitive African landscape sets the scene for this transgression to emerge as Kurtz is relocated away from the enfeebling façade of decayed European civilization and transplanted into the primeval jungle as a test of his strength. As we see, Kurtz both rises and falls accordingly. The appended postscript to Kurtz's report to the Society for the Suppression of Savage Customs, "Exterminate all the brutes!" (2008, 83), signals a clear break from, and abandonment of any pretense to observe, the bounds of Christian charity and notions of progress. As Marlow tells us, "I had to deal with a being to whom I could not appeal to in the name of anything high or low" (111). The ambivalence that Marlow feels toward Kurtz seems clearly to reflect Conrad's own ambivalence toward Nietzschean philosophy.

Importantly, the construction of Kurtz seems not just indebted to Nietzschean thought but to the historical personage of Nietzsche himself, as Alexander notes the parallels between the philosopher and Conrad's creation of the megalomaniacal character whose "soul ... alone in the wilderness . . . had looked within itself . . . and gone mad" (1980, 111). It was well known that Nietzsche, with his iconoclast brilliance and multifold talents for art, music, and oratory (similar to those possessed by the fictional Kurtz) had taken the intellectual world by storm but that his career ended suddenly when he suffered a complete mental and physical collapse and that "he ha[d] gone out of his mind" as the publication the *Academy* put it in 1898 (qtd. in Alexander 1980, 99). Conrad shows awareness of this in an 1899 letter to Edward Garnett regarding popular response to an article Garnett had written about Nietzschean philosophy. When he writes, "I've had letters about your Nietzsche from all sorts of people. You have stirred some brains! I don't think there's anything wrong with *your* wits!" (1989, vol. 2, 209; original emphasis), Conrad seems to be referencing Nietzsche's deteriorated mental state.

Alexander cites contemporary response to translations in English of Nietzsche's work that show, for example, a belief that in Nietzsche "the intensity of self was an obsession; and from a burning desire to preach the divine right of self-hood—if you will, of selfishness—he fell into that unimaginable state in which oneself becomes the universe, and the mind has burst its barriers" (qtd. in Alexander 1980, 108–9). The belief that the provocative egotistical strain in Nietzsche's thoughts was responsible for a madness that is solipsistic in nature is reflected in the depiction of Kurtz as the exuberant egotist whose collapse seems a direct consequence of his transgression against convention and altruism, his will to power. After listening to the harlequin sing Kurtz's praises while at the same time cataloging his unhinged behavior, Marlow declares in response, "Why! He's mad" (2008, 94). When he later makes the distinction between

Kurtz's intelligence and his soul, he describes him as *not* "a lunatic," that "his intelligence was perfectly clear—concentrated, it is true, upon himself with horrible intensity" (111). The spectacle of the mounted human heads turned inward provide the perfect metaphor for this Nietzschean "intensity of self" and what Marlow declares as "the inconceivable mystery of a soul that knew no restraint, no faith, no fear" (111).

While his contemporaries referenced Nietzsche's mental state in terms of his personality and saw it perhaps as a consequence of the peculiar nature of his intellectual work, even a poetically just natural culmination of his philosophical trajectory of defiance, speculation arose as to the true nature of his affliction. The hypothesis that he suffered from syphilis was advanced and debated throughout the twentieth century. Deborah Hayden (2004) outlines the case for a syphilis diagnosis, while Leonard Sax (2003) concluded that he suffered from cancer. Of course, the actual reason for Nietzsche's collapse is not the important question for our purposes. What matters is the perception. While Sax suggests that the rumor of syphilis was invented in the twentieth century, the paperwork for Nietzsche's admission to the nerve clinic in Basel in 1889 following his collapse indicated "Syphilit. Infect" (Hayden 2004, 174). Correct or not, that this diagnosis was so readily made is not merely a testament to the limited state of medical knowledge (if in fact Sax and other critics are correct) but also to the ubiquity of the disease of syphilis in popular perception. As Sax acknowledges, in such cases of insanity "The diagnosis was always assumed to be 'dementia paralytica'—also known as general paresis of the insane, progressive paralysis, or paretic syphilis—that form of syphilis in which the brain is most affected" (2003, 48). Nietzsche's friend, Franz Overbeck, reported that at the point of his breakdown, Nietzsche

> sang loudly, raving, uttering "bits and pieces from the world of ideas in which he has been living, and also in short sentences, in an indescribably muffled tone, sublime, wonderfully clairvoyant. Unspeakably horrible things would be audible, about himself as the successor of the dead God, the whole thing punctuated, as it were, on the piano, whereupon more convulsions and outbursts would follow." (Hayden 2004, 173–4)

The admitting Dr. Wille, whose expertise was diagnosing paralysis of the insane, interpreted these outbursts as evidence of tertiary syphilis.

The point of conjecture here is whether the general public would also have understood Nietzsche's insanity in the same way and, more specifically, whether Conrad would have come to such a conclusion based on what was generally known about Nietzsche's symptoms. Given the stigma attached to a syphilis diagnosis, it is understandable that friends and family endeavored to keep it a secret. Nietzsche's sister in particular worked to maintain the secrecy. And for the same reason, we would not expect to see public conjecture in the printed record naming syphilis as a source for Nietzsche's aggrandizing madness. But as Elaine Showalter points out in her foundational work on syphilis and literature, men were as a rule very acquainted with the symptoms of the disease:

> In the Victorian home, handbooks of popular medicine made images of the syphilitic wages of premarital and extramarital sin available for the instruction of the young boy. . . . As a result of this publicity, and because anxieties about syphilis were so intense, Victorian nerve specialists complained of rampant syphilophobia among their male patients. . . . the male syphilophobic fantasy drew on the guilty acknowledgment of a monstrous sexual self. The disease was the eruption of a repressed desire, the surfacing of a secret life. (1990, 92–93)

As early as 1902, the neurologist and psychiatrist PJ Mobius declared, after his examination of the medical records, that Nietzsche was indeed a syphilitic whose symptoms predated his 1889 collapse, claiming, according to Hayden, that "Only those who are intellectually deaf . . . can miss the undertones of progressive [syphilitic] paralysis in *Thus Spoke Zarathustra*" (2004, 180–181). Likewise, Freud also considered Nietzsche's diagnosis to be undisputedly tertiary syphilis and acknowledged as much in 1908, stating, "It is the loosening process resulting from paresis that gave him the capacity for the quite extraordinary achievement of seeing through all layers and recognizing the instincts at the very base" (qtd. in Hayden 2004, 177).

While Mobius's and Freud's insights postdate *Heart of Darkness*, we can assume that Conrad was not "intellectually deaf" to the symptoms of Nietzsche's madness that seemed to have inspired his creation of Kurtz. Although explainable by "jungle fever," a concept that was "a product of racist Victorian medico-anthropological theories" (Roger 2012, 30),

Kurtz's descent into insanity also might be seen by Conrad as manifestations of the feared "Great Imitator," as syphilis was also known, given "its facility in mimicking many other conditions" (Hayden 2004, xvi) and given that the true cause of syphilis was not discovered until 1906.[9] Such slipperiness is consistent with the long acknowledged evasiveness of Conrad's prose, what Achebe referred to as "stylistic flaw" (2006, 337) as well as the many instances in which Marlow claims to be unable to put his finger on exactly what he wishes to say, such as when he frustratedly proclaims to who he imagines are his incredulous or unsympathetic auditors, "This is the worst of trying to tell. … Here you all are, each moored with two good addresses . . ." (Conrad 2008, 78). He also references and questions his ability to have seen the significance of something at the time, such as the wrecking of the steamer: "I did not see the real significance of that wreck at once. I fancy I see it now, but I am not sure—not at all" (32). This ineffability that characterizes the narrative also characterizes the discourse surrounding syphilis diagnosis.

As we have seen, critics have long acknowledged the idea of Nietzsche and his philosophies as a source for the creation of Kurtz. The feature of Kurtz's conduct and personality that most notably link him with Nietzsche and syphilis is the brilliant euphoria that appears to have preceded his collapse. The quote from Freud cited above in reference to Nietzsche might equally be a description of Kurtz as attested to in the novella by the harlequin and others. Kurtz's ability to see through "the layers" and see "the instincts at the very base" is precisely what Marlow finds so admirable about him—exactly what seduces him, as it were: "Although Marlow is horrified by Kurtz's insanity, he also recognizes that [he] . . . has gained access to a deeper truth of self-knowledge" (Roger 2012, 57). The clarity and directness represented by Kurtz is a refreshing and attractive counterpoint to the murkiness that characterizes Marlow's attempts at delineating perspective.

In her location of *Heart of Darkness* in the Victorian medical discourse surrounding tropical disease, Charlotte Roger, while acknowledging that insanity and warm climates go hand in hand in the European literary imagination, makes the observation that "Conrad's fiction is unique, however, in positing that 'logic' exists in the delirium of those who go mad in the tropics" (2012, 40). She further states, "The notion that madness and moral depravity afford the insane insights that debunk conventional thought is a dominant theme in both 'An Outpost of Progress' and *Heart of Darkness*" (41), but Roger doesn't account for why Conrad should distinguish himself in this regard other than to say that this feature of his work forms a part of his modernist style. An answer to the question of this uniqueness can be found in expanding our model for Kurtz's disease to include not just tropical disorders but those associated with bodily, or perhaps more specifically, venereal transmission. As we have seen, a pivotal part of Nietzsche's syphilis diagnosis stemmed from the exuberance and euphoria found in his writing prior to his collapse. Indeed, his genius was seen by some to be a result of his illness as understood in the following description:

> Right before madness, the syphilitic was often rewarded, in a kind of Faustian bargain for enduring the pain and despair, by episodes of creative euphoria, electrified, joyous energy when grandiosity led to new vision. The heightened perception, dazzling insights, and almost mystical knowledge experienced during this time were expressed while precision of form was still possible. At the end of the nineteenth century, it was believed that, in rare instances, syphilis could produce a genius. (Hayden 2004, xvii)

Kurtz, as we are told over and over again, is an exception, a remarkable man, and the description of his genius as well as his collapse are consistent with this nineteenth-century understanding that links the disease with remarkable vision. As Marlow says, Kurtz's insight was "an affirmation, a moral victory paid for by innumerable defeats, by abominable terrors" (Conrad 2008, 119). "This man has enlarged my mind (90)," the harlequin tells us, "We talked of everything . . . Everything! Everything! (92)" and later, "'Oh! I'll never, never meet such a man again. You ought to have heard him recite poetry— his own, too, it was, he told me. Poetry!' He rolled his eyes at the recollection of these delights. 'Oh, he enlarged my mind!'" he repeats. Just before his final collapse, Kurtz tells Marlow, "I had immense plans . . . I was on the threshold of great things" (110). Just as Nietzsche's work served for many as a guide to transcend the shallowness of bourgeois morality, Marlow's time with Kurtz and his grandiloquence allow Marlow to come to resent "the sight of people hurrying through the street to filch a little money from each other, to devour their infamous cookery, to gulp their unwholesome beer, to dream their insignificant and silly dreams" (119).

The report for the International Society for the Suppression of Savage Customs also reads like a paresis-inspired piece of eloquence, according to Marlow. "It was eloquent, vibrating with eloquence, but too high-strung, I think. Seventeen pages of close writing he had found time for! But this must have been before his—let us say—nerves, went wrong . . . . But it was a beautiful piece of writing" (82). Characteristically, Marlow invokes secrecy when he hedges with his euphemism about "nerves" to use the phrase, "let us say." The question that hangs over this work is why and what Marlow or Conrad finds so unsayable. Indeed, Conrad sets up this secret as a Victorian gothic puzzle that deliberately obfuscates the harsh, repressed realities that underwrite the culture's great progressive claims. Consider this passage:

> And for a moment it seemed to me as if I also were buried in a vast grave full of unspeakable secrets. I felt an intolerable weight oppressing my breast, the smell of the damp earth, the unseen presence of victorious corruption, the darkness of an impenetrable night.... The Russian tapped me on the shoulder. I heard him mumbling and stammering something about 'brother seaman—couldn't conceal— knowledge of matters that would affect Mr. Kurtz's reputation.' I waited. For him evidently Mr. Kurtz was not in his grave; I suspect that for him Mr. Kurtz was one of the immortals. "Well!" said I at last, "speak out. As it happens, I am Mr. Kurtz's friend—in a way." (104–105)

Certainly, the colonial Congo and acts committed there are sites of shame, but as Roberts has pointed out, given that Marlow is willing to narrate the horror of the impaled human heads, what could be so much more appalling that requires him to resort to vague allusions and secrecy? Roberts reads this secrecy as evidence of the homoerotic closet, saying that it evokes "the homophobic taboo of 'love that dare not speak its name'" (2000, 133). But as we have seen, the stigma of syphilis also required the same closeting. Indeed, in the passage quoted above, the handling of Kurtz's "secret" resembles the handling of Nietzsche's: friends and family endeavored to protect the philosopher's reputation.

Besides his unhinged brilliance, Kurtz exhibits other features of the disease. Using contemporary racist stereotypes from medical and social science, Conrad creates a character who has, for all intents and purposes, "gone native," and, on one level, the story insists on a connection between Kurtz's despicable crimes and his having deteriorated into a primitive state that is the antithesis of the cultured European. Theories of social Darwinism and unilinear cultural evolution with its stages of savagery and barbarism are at work not only in Conrad's imagining of the Congo and its people but in his evocation of Kurtz as having fallen victim to primitive degeneracy. This is significant in the current context given the association in eugenics science between syphilis and degeneracy. For example, in his review of a book on the subject, Eugene S. Talbot specifically cites syphilis as one of the known leading causes of degeneracy and catalogs the types of "stigmata" associated with the condition, which include "intellectual degeneracy, such as paranoia, hysteria, epilepsy, idiocy, and one-sided genius" as well as "ethical degeneracy" and its component characteristics of "crime, prostitution, pauperism, and inebriety" (qtd. in Patrick 1899, 372).

In addition, Kurtz shows some of the very marked physical traits associated with syphilis and its progression. Marlow tells us that Kurtz's head was bald: "this— ah—specimen, was impressively bald. The wilderness had patted him on the head, and, behold, it was like a ball— an ivory ball; it had caressed him, and—lo!—he had withered; it had taken him, loved him, embraced him, got into his veins, consumed his flesh, and sealed his soul to its own by the inconceivable ceremonies of some devilish initiation" (Conrad 2008, 79). Kurtz's "withering" and baldness are etiologically linked to the "devilish initiation" that has brought on his affliction, and it is hard to ignore the erotically inflected language of Marlow's prose here. While the bald head of Kurtz links him with ivory, baldness was also associated with syphilis, both as a symptom of the disease and its treatments with mercury.[10] Furthermore, Kurtz's inability to walk also signifies the paralysis of tertiary syphilis. Marlow tells us, "He can't walk—he is crawling on all-fours" (108). Kurtz's motor impairment here is reminiscent perhaps of Rudyard Kipling's depiction of the character Tighe in the 1893 short story, "Love-o'-Women," to which Kipling attributes the affliction of tabes dorsalis or syphilitic myelopathy, a weakening of the nerves that can impair the ability to walk. According to Vora and Lyons (2004), Kipling "accurately describes the clinical syndrome of tabes dorsalis-- popularly known as locomotor ataxia at that time. . . . The diagnosis of 'Locomotus attacks us' seemed well known. . . Kipling seems aware of the association between sexual promiscuity, syphilis, and locomotor ataxia." There is also an indication that Kurtz (like Nietzsche) had developed difficulty seeing as he appears unable to detect the light of a candle a foot away from him.

While the symptoms of Kurtz's illness are consistent with syphilis, there is another dimension of the narrative that further situates it within nineteenth-century syphilis discourse. Doctors faced a particular dilemma in confronting their patients with a syphilis diagnosis given the stigmatized nature of the disease. The secrecy surrounding the disease extended into medical practice with physicians uncertain about their ethical obligations with regard to disclosure about patients' medical conditions. According to Nicholas Jabbour (2000), in America, "it was not always clear if a doctor should even tell a patient that he had syphilis." D.W. Cathell in 1882 expressed this concern to his colleagues. His statement exemplifies the ambivalence and anxiety experienced by physicians in confronting the diagnosis as well as the moralistic ideology surrounding sexually transmitted disease that required evasion even within the scientifically minded medical community. "Even when you are positive that a person has syphilis, it is not always best to say so. Prudence will sometimes require you to reserve your opinion, but at the same time give the proper medicine. Indeed, in practising medicine, you will see and understand many *sins* and *blemishes* of which you must appear oblivious" (qtd. in Jabbour 2000; emphasis added).

Middle class women's relationship to syphilis was perhaps a particularly tragic one, as they were typically infected by their husbands and often unknowingly. While medical ethics required patient confidentiality, many doctors experienced the question about whether to warn unsuspecting women about the likelihood of infection as a dilemma, particularly in cases of engaged couples when the doctor knew that the husband was infected and that the woman was about to, in effect, marry into the disease: "Many [American] physicians felt as though they were accomplices in a crime by not informing innocent women of the medical condition of their future husbands. . . . The classic example was a case in which an innocent young woman was about to make a grave error by unknowingly marrying a syphilitic without a moral conscience" (Jabbour 2000). Physicians were divided on the question of whether to disclose and breach confidentiality or maintain privacy at all costs, and they seemed to experience the issue as a profound and urgent moral crisis, as suggested by the anonymous quotes that Jabbour supplies to illustrate the seriousness of the ethical question, quotes which he describes as "colorful" to suggest the heart-felt positions of both sides. One physician who was in favor of informing the woman saw it as a kind of civil disobedience. "[S]hall we respond with a silence which may be misunderstood and thus render ourselves accomplices of the fruits of which will be so deplorable? Never would I have the courage to obey the law under such circumstances. My conscience would speak higher than it." Another doctor, who found the idea of breaking silence abhorrent, declared: "It [is] treason, perpetrated with the '*best intentions*,' but still a treason, for [the patients are] no longer masters of the secret which no doubt would not have been revealed if they had known what use was going to be made of it" (Jabbour 2000; emphasis added).

Showalter substantiates that wives who became sick invariably contracted the disease from their promiscuous husbands "with almost unfailing regularity," so much so that "One popular manual of venereology gave instructions to the doctor on breaking the bad news to a syphilitic wife" (1990, 94). This dilemma—about how much should be revealed to women and how much the husband's privacy should be respected—is reflected in the final scene of *Heart of Darkness* with Kurtz's fiancée, the Intended. Marlow acts the part of the doctor caught in the bind of confidentiality and decorum that physicians found themselves in with regard to affianced couples. Indeed the melodramatic character of Marlow's diction throughout the narrative matches the "colorful" tone of the physicians' comments cited above, and the physicians' comments themselves seem to capture the essential moral quandary that Marlow finds himself in at narrative's end about whether he should compromise himself by becoming complicit in a crime through his silence or whether he should break the rugged code of masculinist allegiance by revealing the truth of

Kurtz's depravity. As in the case of the doctor treating the syphilitic husband, each option is ethically tainted and neither is fully satisfactory.

The impossibly good and chaste Intended, so good as to provoke Marlow's infamous comment "the women . . . are out of it" (Conrad 2008, 79) altogether, fits the bill of the innocent wife/fiancee who is victim to secret sexual forces that she cannot control. The synecdochal image of the Intended's "forehead, smooth and white, [that] remained illumined by the inextinguishable light of belief and love" (126) identifies her as the preserver of marital fidelity and domesticity, "that great and saving illusion" (127), that the worldly promiscuous husband has darkly violated. Marlow is tasked with breaking to her the truth of "the horned shapes" (a sexually charged image) and "the abject pleading, his abject threats" and "the colossal scale of his vile desires" (123). But instead Marlow elects to preserve Kurtz's confidentiality and remain loyal to his "choice of nightmares": "I remained to dream the nightmare out to the end, and to show my loyalty to Kurtz once more" (117).[11] Marlow is in the same impossible situation as the ethical physician who must choose between honoring two competing sacred principles.

By choosing to honor privacy, Marlow also elects to participate in the continued shrouding of the dark side of desire that becomes emblematic of a homosocial allegiance undergirding both domestic violation of women as well as the expansion of the colonial enterprise and its human and environmental devastations, both late Victorian practices shrouded in secrecy ripe for rendering through the discourse of syphilis. While Marlow in this scene may convince himself he is protecting the delicate sensibilities of the Intended, he is in fact depriving her of the truth and the necessary grounds to "divorce" herself from the memory of Kurtz (as syphilis was a legal grounds for dissolving actual marriages). Thus Marlow's mercy, his "good intentions" as it were, (the Intended's name, which suggests this phrase, echoes the language of the physician's argument for silence cited above), in actuality functions as a potent means of maintaining patriarchal control over women's lives as well as a mechanism to continue the exploitation of the Congo. Marlow's role then is analogous to that of the reticent physician's; he becomes accomplice to a crime in an effort to uphold a conflicted ethical claim. This complicity haunting Marlow resonates with that feared by nineteenth-century syphilis doctors who resented their role as arbiters of fate.

To identify the projection of syphilis in *Heart of Darkness* is in no way to diminish the power of the work or reduce it to a pedestrian concern of syphiliphobia. Rather, it is a testament to the seriousness of the disease and its cultural importance that Conrad would, knowingly or unknowingly, enshrine this discourse in this most important metaphysical work. Indeed there is a brilliant deployment here of this rhetoric of disease to yoke together medical fears and problematic sexual morality besetting a culture with revelation of and commentary about a global violence infecting self-congratulatory European benevolence and charity. The syphilis paradigm seems to provide a perfect vehicle for achieving this fictive exploration. Thus, reading *Heart of Darkness* as a syphilis narrative serves to remind us of what may now be easy to forget: the significance of the potent, silent anxiety that informed lives and literature at century's end and how it shaped the world.

Notes

1. Conrad's use of women characters also fits with Showalter's schema for the pervasive presence of syphilis in *fin de siècle* literature: By the 1890s the syphilitic male had become an arch-villain of feminist protest fiction, a carrier of contamination and madness, and a threat to the spiritual evolution of the human race. In men's writing of the period, however, women are the enemies, whether as the femmes fatales who lure men into sexual temptation only to destroy them, the frigid wives who drive them to the brothels, or the puritanical women novelists, readers, and reviewers who would emasculate their art (1990, 88).
2. While Roberts and others read this as evidence of same-sex desire, it is of course possible to read it as masculine appropriation and trivialization of the feminized discourse of love. Marlow's "amusement" at the prospect of Kurtz and the Russian discussing love can equally suggest that it is not a sufficiently masculine topic worthy of discussion between men about ideals. Thus, the Russian hastens to add the adverb "generally," to suggest it was an abstraction worthy of philosophical engagement.

3. See Alexander (1980) for a discussion of the relationship between Rimbaud and Verlaine as a model for the Kurtz/harlequin relationship.
4. Watts's (2012) analysis focuses on the *Blackwood's Magazine* text published in 1899 under the title "*The* Heart of Darkness" (our emphasis).
5. This passage about the reanimated dead with its emphasis on Kurtz's height—that he was at least 7 feet tall—also suggests Mary Shelley's *Frankenstein*, especially when we consider it in light of the "whited sepulcher" motif and Marlow's assertion that "all Europe contributed to the making of Kurtz" (Conrad 2008, 81–82). As such, Kurtz is assembled from the metaphorical charnel house of European culture's degeneration in the same way Frankenstein's progeny was produced from parts of forsaken corpses.
6. The inward facing heads suggest a metaphor for the madness of tertiary syphilis that is reinforced by Marlow's description of Kurtz's soul, "But his soul was mad. Being alone in the wilderness, it had looked within itself, and, by heavens! I tell you, it had gone mad" (Conrad 2008, 111). It is also another moment in the story where appearances from a distance are deceptive, and it is not until Marlow takes a closer look that he understands that the harmless looking objects are abominations. This process interestingly parallels the deceptive nature of the disease of syphilis that is elusive in presentation and manifestation.
7. One of Conrad's letters in Volume 8 indicates a more than cursory acquaintance with the details of Columbus's voyages as he invokes the name of "Pinzon" (sic) in humorous analogy. Pinzon was the captain of the *Nina* on the first voyage (Conrad 1986, 48).
8. As the Russian harlequin tells us, "There hasn't been a drop of medicine or a mouthful of invalid food for months here. He was shamefully abandoned. A man like this, with such ideas" (Conrad 2008, 98).
9. Despite its association with illicit sexual activity, because syphilis transmission was not entirely understood, the erroneous belief that syphilis was passed onto the child through the father's sperm was entertained by many and thus raised the specter of a hereditary possibility for the disease, a situation that evoked fears of degeneracy. *Heart of Darkness* is obviously deeply enmeshed in the discourse of degeneracy.
10. Interestingly, according to N.F. Lowe, the connection between syphilis and madness was not established until the nineteenth century, and prior to that madness and sex were linked through the concept of excessive stimulation. A shaved head could help "cool the brain and relieve the

pressure caused by overstimulation." According to William Battie's 1758 *Treatise on Madness*, the "endless thinking" engaged in by what Battie termed "infirm and shattered philosophers" was also a source of madness (qtd. in Lowe 1996, 181).

11. Marlow references the idea of a choice of nightmares in three other instances (104,108,114).

References

Achebe, Chinua. 2006. An Image of Africa. In *Heart of Darkness: Norton Critical Edition*, ed. Paul B. Armstrong, 4th ed., 336–349. New York: Norton.

Alexander, George B. 1980. In Search of the Real Mr. Kurtz: A Study of Multiple Sources in Conrad's *Heart of Darkness*. Dissertation, New York University.

Anonymous. (1888) 2009. *My Secret Life*. http://www.gutenberg.org/files/30360/30360-h/30360-h.htm

Arrizabalaga, Jon, John Henderson, and Roger French. 1997. *The Great Pox: The French Disease in Renaissance Europe*. New Haven: Yale University Press.

Billy, Theodore. 1997. *A Wilderness of Words: Closure and Disclosure in Conrad's Short Fiction*. Lubbock: Texas Tech University Press.

Butte, George. 1989. What Silenus Knew: Conrad's Uneasy Debt to Nietzsche. *Comparative Literature* 41 (2): 155–169.

Conrad, Joseph. 1926. Geography and Some Explorers. In *Last Essays*, 1–31. London: J.M. Dent & Sons.

———. 1986. *The Collected Letters*, ed. Frederick R. Karl and Laurence Davies, vols. 2–8. Cambridge: Cambridge University Press.

———. (1902) 2008. *Heart of Darkness*. Ebook.http://www.planetebook.com/ebooks/Heart-of-Darkness.pdf

Crow, Charles L. 2009. *American Gothic*. Cardiff: University of Wales Press.

Davidson, Roger, and Lesley A. Hall. 2001. Introduction. In *In Sex, Sin and Suffering: Venereal Disease and European Society since 1870*, ed. Roger Davidson and Lesley A. Hall. London: Routledge.

Greaney, Michael. 2002. *Conrad, Language, and Narrative*. Cambridge: Cambridge University Press.

Hayden, Deborah. 2004. *Pox: Genius, Madness, and the Mysteries of Syphilis*. New York: Basic.

Jabbour, Nicholas. 2000. Syphilis from 1880 to 1920: A Public Health Nightmare and the First Challenge to Medical Ethics. *Essays in History* 42. Web.

Lowe, N.F. 1996. The Meaning of Venereal Disease in Hogarth's Graphic Art. In *The Secret Malady: Venereal Disease in Eighteenth Century Britain and France*, ed. Linda E. Merians, 168–182. Lexington: University Press of Kentucky.

Mitchell, Jonathan, and Michael O'Rourke. 2011. Quempire: A Loiterly Journey into Heart of Darkness. *Thamyris Intersecting* 22: 75–96.

Paris, Bernard. 2005. *Conrad's Charlie Marlow: A New Approach to "Heart of Darkness" and Lord Jim*. New York: Palgrave.

Patrick, G.T.W. 1899. Review of *Degeneracy: Its Causes, Signs ,and Results*, by Eugene S. Talbot. *Science* 9 (January–June): 372–373.

Renner, Stanley W. 2012. *The Secret Sharer*, Nietzsche, and Conrad's New Man. *Conradiana* 44 (2–3): 145–146.

Roberts, Andrew Michael. 2000. *Conrad and Masculinity*. New York: Palgrave.

Roger, Charlotte. 2012. *Jungle Fever: Exploring Madness and Medicine in Twentieth-century Tropical Narratives*. Nashville: University of Vanderbilt Press.

Ruppel, Richard. 2008. *Homosexuality in the Life and Work of Joseph Conrad*. New York: Routledge.

Said, Edward. 1979. *Orientalism*. New York: Vintage.

Sax, Leonard. 2003. What Was the Cause of Nietzsche's Dementia? *Journal of Medical Biography* 11: 47–54.

Showalter, Elaine. 1990. Syphilis. Sexuality, and the Fiction of the Fin de Siecle. In *Sex, Politics, and Science in the Nineteenth Century Novel*, ed. Ruth Bernard Yeazell, 89–115. Baltimore: Johns Hopkins University Press.

Stape, John. 2007. *The Several Lives of Joseph Conrad*. New York: Pantheon.

Vaughan, Megan. 1991. *Curing their Ills: Colonial Power and African Illness*. Stanford: Stanford University Press.

Vora, Set K., and Robert W. Lyons. 2004. The Medical Kipling—Syphilis, Tabes Dorsalis, and Romber's Test. *Emerging Infectious Diseases* 10(6).

Wasson, Sara. 2014. Gothic Cities and Suburbs, 1800–present. In *The Gothic World*, ed. Glennis Byron and Dale Townshend, 132–142. New York: Routledge.

Watts, Cedric. 2012. Conradian Eldritch: Bram Stoker's *Dracula* and Joseph Conrad's 'The Heart of Darkness'. *Conradian* 37 (2): 1–18.

"Everybody Has It": Syphilis and the Human Condition in the Writings of Ernest Hemingway

Lisa Tyler

As the son of an obstetrician (Sanford 1999, 112), Ernest Hemingway probably knew better than many men of his generation about the horrific consequences of sexually transmitted diseases. One biographer speculates that the young Ernest was horrified by "the horrible color plates in [his father] Ed's medical books that showed chancres and venereal ulcers" (Meyers 1985, 199). References to venereal disease pepper Hemingway's writings, from his early poetry and "A Very Short Story" (first published in 1924) to "Fathers and Sons" (1933) and the posthumously published *Under Kilimanjaro* (written in the 1950s). Hemingway also refers to syphilis in *The Sun Also Rises* (1926), *A Farewell to Arms* (1929), *Death in the Afternoon* (1932), "One Reader Writes" (1933), *To Have and Have Not* (1937), *Across the River and into the Trees* (1950), *A Moveable Feast* (1964, posthumously), *Islands in the Stream* (1970, posthumously), and his correspondence. Yet despite the plethora of references to sexually transmitted diseases, discussions of Hemingway's representations of these illnesses are rare.[1] In fact, there are remarkably few discussions of the

L. Tyler (✉)
Sinclair Community College, Dayton, OH, USA

K. Nixon, L. Servitje (eds.), *Syphilis and Subjectivity*,
https://doi.org/10.1007/978-3-319-66367-8_8

significance of syphilis in modernist literature in general.[2] In this chapter, I want to unpack the cultural relevance of these various references to venereal disease in Hemingway's writings and examine the cultural work that syphilitic discourse performs in his fiction.

The very mention of any form of venereal disease in his writings signals Hemingway's commitment to literary modernism and the shock of the new. Syphilis, the life-long, potentially fatal illness for which there was no permanent remedy until 1943, became a trope for Hemingway. Again and again, he presents sexually transmitted diseases in general, and syphilis in particular, as the universal human condition. Hemingway sees syphilis as both a concrete medical reality of his time and an iconic form of human suffering, a metaphor for what all humans must eventually endure: suffering for which there is, indeed, no remedy. And he explicitly links that suffering both to unreasonable and inherently dangerous societal expectations for masculine behavior and to the emotional pain of the depression he repeatedly experienced.

No analysis of syphilis in Hemingway's writings would be complete without a discussion of the flash fiction "One Reader Writes," first published in *Winner Take Nothing* (1933). In this haunting story, a veteran's wife writes a plaintive letter to a medical columnist in the newspaper asking for advice on whether she can safely resume marital relations with a husband undergoing treatment for syphilis. She is not an educated woman—she admits she doesn't know how to spell the name of the disease and so spells it phonetically as "sifilus"—and she isn't sure which of the male authorities in her life to trust: her husband, who insists he will no longer be contagious after his treatment is completed; her father, who says "One could well wish themselves dead if once they became a victim of that malady" (1987, 320); or the physician who writes a medical advice column in the newspaper: "In the picture in the paper he looks like he'd know" (1987, 321).

Ironically, none of these authorities is trustworthy: She fears that her husband is misleading her out of self-interest, and she "dare not ask [her] parents," presumably out of a fear of moral condemnation. The doctor to whom she directs her letter might seem to be an objective authority. But the letter that makes up two-thirds of the story was a real letter received by Dr. Logan Clendening of Kansas City, the author of a syndicated medical column called "Diet and Health" (Baker 1969, 604n). Clendening gave it to Hemingway, a friend of his, along with several other letters. Hemingway altered its location and date, added an introduction and a conclusion, and published it as a short story. While Paul Smith gives a halfhearted defense of the ethics of what he describes as Hemingway's "opportunism" (299), Clendening's decision to share the letter in the first place seems less defensible—although no doubt he would argue that anyone who writes to a newspaper columnist has forfeited her right to privacy.

Interestingly, the letter writer never criticizes her husband for the infidelity that must have preceded his contraction of the disease: "I don't care what he did to get it" (Hemingway 1987, 321). The story evokes an alternative "moral ideology" associated with the disease, an ideology Elaine Showalter identifies in fin de siècle writing:

> For respectable women, syphilis had nothing to do with marital transgression, secret vices, or monstrous desires; it was more likely the wages of ignorance than the wages of sin. . . . Although prostitutes constituted the largest category of female syphilitics and general paralytics, the plight of the diseased wife also generated a potent mythology. (94)

Showalter notes that turn-of-the-century feminists described a vast masculine conspiracy of physicians, lawmakers, and libertines working to protect men from the consequences of their lustful actions, at the expense of innocent women.

Certainly, the unnamed letter writer in Hemingway's story is innocent, even though her husband has carelessly indulged his lust. Her desperate sexual longing is evident in Hemingway's characteristic use of repetition: "It's such a long time though. It's a long time. And it's been a long time. My Christ, it's been a long time" (Hemingway 1987, 321). Unlike her husband, she has evidently not resorted to infidelity during his long naval deployment. But the woman's final appeal is to yet another masculine authority: "I wish to Christ he hadn't got any kind of malady" (321). The importance of this final appeal is underscored by the fact that Hemingway considered "Light from the East" (a reference to Christ, much like "The Light of the World," a painting whose name he used as the ironic title of another short story) as a title for the story (Smith 1989, 298). Calling this story about syphilis "Light from the East" would have been particularly ironic given that the writer's husband contracted the illness in Shanghai—in the Far East. Hemingway suggests here that religious authority—like marital authority, paternal authority, and both medical and journalistic authorities—has little help to offer her. Every source of (masculine, patriarchal) authority fails the letter writer, much as every source of (masculine, patriarchal) authority (including his father, the military, the police, the priesthood, and finally even a king) fails Nick Adams of *In Our Time* (Tyler 2016). If syphilis becomes, for Hemingway, an emblem of the dangers of modernity, this poignant short story suggests that no social authority can help victims of syphilis, of careless masculine risk-taking, of depression, and perhaps even of the evils of modernity cope with their uncertainty, isolation, and mental anguish.

In invoking the taboo subject of syphilis in his fiction, Hemingway is rebelling against his parents' Congregationalist conservatism but also flouting societal standards. His parents were probably typical of their generation in their reaction to *In Our Time*: horrified by their son's choice of subject matter in the 1925 short story collection, they returned all six of their complimentary copies. They were particularly appalled by "A Very Short Story," in which the unnamed protagonist, after being abruptly jilted by a young woman named Luz, contracts gonorrhea (referred to as "the clap") through a hurried sexual encounter with a salesgirl in a Chicago taxi (1925, 66). Hemingway's father wrote to tell him sternly that "no gentleman spoke of venereal disease outside a doctor's office" (Sanford 1999, 219).

So writing about syphilis at all was shocking, new, and quintessentially modern. Even as late as the 1930s, newspapers avoided printing the words "syphilis" and "gonorrhea" so as not to offend the moral sensibilities of their readers (Brandt 1987, 136). As the surgeon general of the United States wrote in a frank, groundbreaking article eventually published in *Reader's Digest* in July 1936, "First and foremost among American handicaps to progress against syphilis is the widespread belief that nice people don't talk about syphilis, nice people don't have syphilis, and nice people shouldn't do anything about those who have syphilis" (quoted in Brandt 1987, 138).

In an apparent contradiction of his earlier commitment to modernism, Hemingway at times echoes this view by depicting venereal disease as a deserved punishment for sexually immoral behavior.[3] Throughout his oeuvre, Hemingway invokes syphilis with physical and moral disgust, as, for example, in *Death in the Afternoon*, where he writes, "I would sooner have the pox than to fall in love with another woman loving the one I have" (1932, 122). In *Death in the Afternoon*, he offers several pages of extended discussion of syphilis, acknowledging that "it is a to-be-expected end, or rather phase, of the life of all fornicators who continue their careers far enough" (101). The use of the term "fornicators" introduces a decidedly biblical undertone to the discussion; Hemingway, raised a Congregationalist (Nickel 2013, 347), at times shared his parents' moral conservatism, noting mockingly that venereal disease serves as a check on immoral sexual behavior: "Within our time the scientists may well abolish these old diseases and we'll live to see the end of all morality" (Hemingway 1932, 104).[4]

Despite this genteel concern, however, there is at least a suggestion that Hemingway later came to view these illnesses (albeit gonorrhea perhaps more than syphilis) more or less as a modern rite of passage, an inevitable part of growing up in modernity. Hemingway himself once bragged to a friend he met during World War II that "he'd 'had the clap' [i.e., gonorrhea] twice before his older friend Bill Smith ever got laid"—a claim for which Scott Donaldson scrupulously notes there is otherwise no biographical evidence whatsoever (1977, 175). Frederic Henry, the protagonist of *A Farewell to Arms* (1929), confesses to Catherine Barkley that he has had a very painful case of gonorrhea, and Catherine, unperturbed, responds, "I wish I'd had it to be like you" (301).

In perhaps the most notable example in Hemingway's literary fiction, in *The Sun Also Rises*, Jake Barnes picks up the prostitute Georgette at the Café Napolitain, and as they cross Paris in a horse-cab, she, unaware of his war wound and its consequences, tries to touch him intimately before he moves her hand away.

> "Never mind."
> "What's the matter? You sick?"
> "Yes."
> "Everybody's sick. I'm sick, too." (Hemingway 1926, 15–16)

Georgette assumes that only a reluctance to transmit disease could explain his resistance to her sexual advances. She goes on to insist a moment later, "It doesn't make any difference with me. It doesn't make any difference with a woman" (Hemingway 1926, 16). Presumably she is willing to risk contagion for the sake of her fee. It is interesting that it is the prostitute[5]—the traditional scapegoat for venereal disease (Brandt 1987, 87)—who introduces the idea that syphilis emblematizes modernity. On one level, her quick reassurance—"Everybody's sick"—emphasizes how widespread and inevitable sexually transmitted diseases have become in 1920s Paris. But on another, it suggests that Hemingway sees this European society as diseased, contaminated, immoral, and permanently damaged by the Great War. It's difficult here not to be reminded of James Joyce's pun in *Ulysses* on "syphilisation" (Joyce 1997, 12.1197). As Allen Brandt notes, "Venereal disease, the palpable evidence of unrestrained sexuality, became a symbol of social disorder and moral decay—a metaphor for evil" (Brandt 1987, 92).[6]

It is perhaps useful here to remember just how prevalent syphilis really was in the early twentieth century: "The admission rate for venereal disease in the Army in 1909 neared 200 per 1,000 men, and one third of all days lost from duty resulted from these infections" (Brandt 1987, 13). As James Joyce observed in a letter to his brother, "I presume there are very few mortals in Europe who are not in danger of waking some morning and finding themselves syphilitic" (quoted in Lyons 1988, 32). The numbers remained high in the general population 20 years later:

> By the early 1930s the most frequently cited figures suggested that approximately one out of every ten Americans suffered from syphilis. Each year, citizens of the United States contracted almost half a million new infections—twice as many cases as tuberculosis and a hundred times the number of cases of the dreaded infantile paralysis [i.e., polio]. (Brandt 1987, 129)

As Jake Barnes's circle in Paris in the mid-1920s included sexually active young people who were mostly American or British, it's reasonable to assume the prevalence of syphilis among them was at least comparable to the rate in the general population in the United States, if not considerably higher.

It is not until *A Farewell to Arms*, however, that an important and sympathetic character in Hemingway's fiction contracts syphilis and undergoes the treatment process typical during World War I. Frederic Henry's friend Rinaldi suffers from both syphilis and its painful treatment with mercury and Salvarsan, both of which Michael Reynolds identifies as "potentially poisonous heavy metals" (Hemingway 1929, 114). Rinaldi describes the initial stages of the disease with clinical accuracy: "'First,' he went on, assuming the manner of a lecturer, 'it's a little pimple. Then we notice a rash between the shoulders. Then we notice nothing at all. We put our faith in mercury'" (1929, 175).

Rinaldi's word choice here suggests that modernity puts its faith in science rather than Christianity, especially as he goes on to verbally abuse the priest. But in this case, at least, Rinaldi's faith in medical science is misplaced, as the medical science of his day offers only a treatment for his illness, not a cure. Hemingway returns to this question in *Across the River and into the Trees*, published in 1950, where he uses the reliability of a medical test for syphilis as a guarantor of his beloved Renata's implicit courage and integrity, which he "knew as absolutely as though he had just read his third Wassermann" (1950, 173). The Wassermann test, developed by August Wassermann in 1906, detects the spirochete in the blood of people infected with the disease (Brandt 1987, 40; Parascandola 2008, 78). At first glance, Hemingway seems to be using this jarring simile to say that the test, like Renata, is infallible—until we consider the word "third," which suggests that medical science is *not* altogether reliable and must be repeatedly checked to ensure certainty. Hemingway also emphasizes in *A Farewell to Arms* the difficulty of simply diagnosing the illness accurately. The major is skeptical of Rinaldi's self-diagnosis: "He thinks . . . he has syphilis. I don't believe it but he may have" (1929, 175). Frederic isn't sure what to think either, telling Catherine later in the novel, "I was wondering whether Rinaldi had the syphilis" (298). Like the woman in "One Reader Writes," Rinaldi cannot rely on the authority of either religious faith or medical science.

It is typical of Hemingway's irony that in *A Farewell to Arms* it is a physician who contracts what at the time was widely viewed as a preventable or at least avoidable illness. "What if I have it?" a drunk and defiant Rinaldi asks when the priest recommends he take leave to recover from the syphilis he has presumably contracted from the prostitutes at the whorehouse he frequents; "Everybody has it. The whole world's got it" (1929, 175). Given the novel's extraordinarily sympathetic portrayal of the diseased surgeon, Rinaldi's comment inscribes his illness as the human condition. As Frederic Henry later tells us, in his bitter diatribe after his son is born dead,

> You did not know what it was about. You never had time to learn. They threw you in and told you the rules and the first time they caught you off base they killed you. Or they killed you gratuitously like Aymo. Or gave you the syphilis like Rinaldi. But they killed you in the end. You could count on that. Stay around and they would kill you. (Hemingway 1929, 327)

Syphilis, like the modern technological warfare that kills Aymo and the modern medical science that cannot save Catherine or her baby, is another inevitable and deadly consequence of modernism.

That might seem like an anachronism, given that in *Death in the Afternoon*, Hemingway describes syphilis with historical inaccuracy as "the disease of the crusaders in the middle ages" (1932, 101). But it is the relative sexual freedom of modernism that causes the disease to spread. He satirically mocks young college graduates whose own foolish behavior gets them into trouble: "They believed [sexual intercourse] was this great new thing that they had just discovered and were most joyously promiscuous until their first experience with disease which they then believed they too had discovered and invented" (102). But there is an underlying seriousness here. Even quite late in his life, Hemingway firmly believed that contracting a sexually transmitted disease was ultimately a failure of personal responsibility: "I was as afraid as the next man in my time and maybe more so. But with the years fear had come to be regarded as a form of stupidity to be classed with overdrafts, acquiring a venereal disease, or eating candies. Fear is a child's vice and while I loved to feel it approach as one does with any vice, it was not for grown men" (2005, 384). The implication is that, like the French writer Guy de Maupassant,[7] who (according to Hemingway) classified venereal disease as a problem of "adolescence" (2005, 102), Hemingway believed that acquiring such an illness was "not for grown men," who were presumably wise enough to know how to avoid contagion.

Not surprisingly, then, Hemingway links the contraction of the ubiquitous venereal disease to careless masculine risk-taking. As the author of a poem improbably titled "Tuberculosis and Syphilis Are the Two Occupational Hazards of the Matador," Hemingway attributes the prevalence of syphilis to an inherent willingness to engage in risky behavior: "Boxers, bullfighters, and soldiers contract syphilis for the same reasons that make them choose those professions. . . . [I]t is a disease of all people who lead lives in which a disregard of consequences dominates" (1932, 100). So in *To Have and Have Not*, for example, World War I veterans discuss prizefighters battling "the old rale," a slang term for syphilis (215). In *Death in the Afternoon*, Hemingway describes the disease (along with tuberculosis, which was then also inflected with overtones of sexual promiscuity) as one of "the occupational diseases" with which matadors must contend (100), and calls it "an industrial accident" (101), just as Rinaldi does in *A Farewell to Arms*: "It's an industrial accident. It's a simple industrial accident" (1929, 175). The term makes it sound as though the disease is a more or less inevitable cost of doing business.[8] If, for Hemingway, masculinity must be proved repeatedly through physical performance in the battlefield, the bullring, the boxing ring, or the bedroom, and the mental requirements for successful physical performance necessarily entail an utter disdain for the consequences (Strychacz 2004), then syphilis becomes an inevitable consequence of (stereotypical) masculinity. Stereotypical expectations for masculine behavior have become, as he suggests in his discussion of the "very severe" masculine hunting ethics he persists in subscribing to in *Under Kilimanjaro*, "too rigid and slightly murderous" (46). Hemingway's syphilitic rhetoric here suggests that modern masculinity is inherently dangerous and life-threatening.

It is in Hemingway's discussion of venereal diseases that he introduces the dictum "There is no remedy for anything in life" (1929, 104). He later adopts it in abbreviated form as a personal motto during his depressive states in *Under Kilimanjaro*, the posthumously published memoir of his second African safari: "No hay remedio," or "There is no remedy," is one of the first phrases Hemingway teaches Debba to say, and he writes, "She thought that it was part of my religion" (2005, 72). She was probably right. Hemingway's fourth wife, Mary, tells him that he used the same expression while talking in his sleep and asks him, "What was it there was no remedy for?" (2005, 71). Hemingway claims he doesn't remember but later insists, "I'm not a no hay remedio boy, really" (72), and Mary responds, "Yes. You are a little bit" but also insists that he is happier now than he was when they met (72).

Interestingly, the phrase *no hay remedio* is an allusion to a painting by Spanish artist Francisco Goya ("Plate 15"), whom Hemingway also describes approvingly in *Death in the Afternoon:*

> Goya did not believe in costume but he did believe in blacks and in grays, in dust and in light, in high places rising from the plains, in the country around Madrid, in movement, in his own cojones, in painting, in etching, and in what he had seen, felt, touched, handled, smelled, enjoyed, drunk, mounted, suffered, spewed-up, lain-with, suspected, observed, loved, hated, lusted, feared, detested, admired, loathed, and destroyed. Naturally no painter has been able to paint all that but he tried. (Hemingway 2005, 205)

Hemingway also name-checks Goya twice in "A Natural History of the Dead," a short story (or, arguably, sketch) embedded in *Death in the Afternoon* (1932, 135, 141). Abundant evidence substantiates the writer's abiding interest in the Romantic painter. Hemingway read two books on Goya, according to Michael Reynolds (1996, 169, 179), and owned at least half a dozen, including three by Goya himself, according to James D. Brasch and Joseph Sigman (1981, 157, 166, 274, 314). According to Miriam B. Mandel (2004, 110), he acquired Goya's two-volume *Tauromaquia* in 1923. He wanted color reproductions of Goya's work to appear in *Death in the Afternoon* (Brand 2004, 165), an ambitious plan scuttled because of the cost involved, but his 1930 article "Bull Fighting, Sport, and Industry" in *Fortune* magazine did include color reproductions of Goya's work (Brand 2004, 183n2).

What is particularly interesting about this connection is that there has long been reason to believe that Goya suffered from syphilis. In 1792, when he was 46, the painter fell seriously ill for several months. His symptoms included dizziness, impaired vision, paralysis, tinnitus, and permanent hearing loss. One of his friends wrote of Goya in a letter, "His lack of reflection has caught up with him, but now we must regard him with the compassion that his disgrace demands, and as a sick man, for whom all remedies must be procured" (quoted in Ravin and Ravin 1999, 166). The comments about Goya's "disgrace" and his "lack of reflection" led to speculation about syphilis as the cause of his symptoms (Hayden 2003, 307). While more recent scholars have suggested various alternative diagnoses, including lead paint poisoning (Felisati and Sperati 2010, 269), Vogt-Koyanagi disease (Cawthorne 1962, 3), and a host of other possibilities (Ravin and Ravin 1999, 166–69), syphilis has never been definitively ruled out. Certainly, Hemingway himself believed syphilis was the cause of Goya's ill health: "Goya's troubles came, mostly, from what he carried between his thighs and they were fairly continuous, very interesting to study, and sometimes seem unnecessary. But the necessary misfortunes we never make ourselves" (Hemingway 1934).

After his mysterious illness, Goya's artistic vision changed dramatically: "Biographers have divided the painting course of Goya into two periods, before and after his illness. The first characterized by joy and light, the second by horror and ghosts" (Felisati and Sperati 2010, 267). "Y no hai remedio" (variously translated as "And there is no help" or "And there's nothing to be done") is the title of Plate 15 in a series of etchings titled *Disasters of War* (*Los Desastres de la Guerra*). Created in 1810, well after Goya's midlife bout of serious illness, this etching depicts one man, blindfolded and with his hands tied to a pole behind him, awaiting his execution while another man lies dead at his feet, already killed by the firing squad visible in the background. It is easy to see why Hemingway, who wrote about executions in *In Our Time*, *A Farewell to Arms*, and *For Whom the Bell Tolls*, would have been drawn to "Y no hai remedio." He also writes in *Death in the Afternoon*, in what seems to be a direct reference to that etching, "But in the case of an execution by a firing squad, or a hanging, . . . if these very simple things were to be made permanent, as, say, Goya tried to make them in *Los Desastros de la Guerra,* it could not be done with any shutting of the eyes" (2015, 3). Obviously he was attracted by Goya's willingness to look at human violence without flinching, and Goya's title phrase, "Y no hai remedio," with its medical implications of incurable illness and psychological implications of unresolvable despair, held a certain resonance for Hemingway.[9] Hemingway's syphilitic rhetoric, then—his repeated invocation of the talismanic Spanish phrase "Y no hai remedio"—becomes a way to externalize the mental anguish of his bouts with depression. It's also reasonable to assume that Hemingway, plagued by mood swings from his twenties onward (Hays 1995) and worried after 1929 that he might commit suicide as his father had, might have been especially unnerved by an incurable physical illness that could end in madness.

Perhaps that explains why, later in his writing career, hopeless cases of venereal disease particularly seemed to haunt Hemingway. Thomas Hudson, an autobiographical character in the posthumously published novel *Islands in the Stream*, despairs at the wretched conditions he witnesses in Cuba: "I drink against poverty, dirt, four-hundred-year-old dust, the nose-snot of children, cracked palm fronds, roofs made from hammered tins, *the shuffle of untreated syphilis*, sewage in the old beds of brooks, lice on the bare necks of infested poultry, scale on the backs of old men's necks, the smell of old women, and the full-blast radio, he thought" (Hemingway 1972, 231–32; emphasis added). Hemingway told Maxwell Perkins that he was rewriting this manuscript in 1947 (1981, 616), when antibiotics such as penicillin could cure more than 90 percent of cases of syphilis (Brandt 1987, 172), so the persistence of *untreated* syphilis cases would have been especially disturbing to a doctor's son. There is also reason to believe that Hemingway blamed venereal disease for his wife Mary's infertility and consequent inability to have the daughter he had long wanted (Burwell 1996, 50; Fuentes 1984, 416)—another reason for him to associate syphilis with depression and find untreated cases particularly saddening.

In *The Sun Also Rises*, Jake Barnes observes that "The bill always came" (Hemingway 1926, 148). For Hemingway, syphilis always represented the inevitable bill to be paid for sexual irresponsibility, but it also represented a larger and existential evil of modernity, a problem he associated with the inherent dangers of performative masculinity and the mental anguish of untreated depression. Traditional sources of authority are no longer trustworthy in modernity, as "One Reader Writes" tells us again and again, and they have no practical solutions to offer anyway. Syphilis, the then-incurable illness that could threaten one's sanity and life, became for Hemingway the perfect trope for the universal human condition in the modern age.

Notes

1. The only extended discussion of venereal disease in Hemingway's work that I have been able to find is Yasushi Takano's (n.d.) essay "Against the Victorian Normalization of Sexuality: A Study of Hemingway's Representation of Syphilis," although Debra A. Moddelmog briefly mentions the social hygiene movement and "Hemingway's resistance to social hygiene morality" in her discussion "Sex, Sexuality, and Marriage" in *Ernest Hemingway in Context* (2013, 360). Mark Spilka briefly discusses Hemingway's angry response to James Jones, who in *From Here to Eternity* had publicly disputed Hemingway's contention, in *Death in the Afternoon*, that venereal diseases are the occupational diseases of soldiers (1990, 114–16). Hemingway seems to have particularly resented Jones's implication that Hemingway didn't know what he was talking about: "From the time I was a kid I had to distinguish between soft and hard chancres and courageous Jones comes along and says *he* had had the clap and it was horrible" (1981, 724–25).
2. See, for example, Fiorenzo Iuliano's "Staging the Stigma: Syphilis and Its Metaphors in Claude McKay's *The Clinic*," Gerard M. Sweeney's note "Wharton's *Bewitched*," Laurence M. Porter's "Syphilis as Muse in Thomas Mann's *Doctor Faustus*," and Thomas Rütten's "Genius and Degenerate? Thomas Mann's *Doktor Faustus* and a Medical Discourse on Syphilis." The sole exception is James Joyce; scholars have discussed at length the significance of syphilis in Joyce's life and work. Kathleen Ferris argues that Joyce had syphilis and that it heavily influenced his fiction: "The evidence, both biographical and literary, that Joyce himself suffered from syphilis is massive" (1995, 124). See also Deborah Hayden (2003, 239–50) and Kevin Birmingham: "James Joyce was going blind because he had syphilis" (2014, 289). For a strongly argued dissent (if not, in my view, on ultimately persuasive one), see J. B. Lyons (1998, especially the collection's title essay, 20–39): "Was he syphilitic? The question, I suspect, is ill-mannered and because those who pose it seem determined to prove that Joyce suffered either from congenital or acquired syphilis, or preferably both, I am glad to say he had neither" (21, Lyons's italics). Ferris notes that Lyons, a Dublin physician, was related to Joyce by marriage (1995, 5). For discussions of allusions to the disease in Joyce's fiction, see Burton A. Waisbren and Florence L. Walzl, Martin Bock, Marian Eide, David Kadlec (90-121), and Michael Timins.

3. Harold Loeb, generally acknowledged as the inspiration for the character of Robert Cohn in *The Sun Also Rises*, has said of Hemingway, "He made himself out to be a sort of bad boy; he certainly wasn't. He was a bit of a Puritan, if anything" (Brian 1988, 48). Yasushi Takano makes a similar point with respect to Hemingway's fiction, arguing that his works "are marked by an equivocalness oscillating between a repugnance for the Victorian moral standard, on the one hand, and an unintentional compliance with it, on the other" (n.d., 2); I believe, however, that Hemingway was more aware of his own ambivalence than Takano gives him credit for.
4. Hemingway wasn't alone in expressing this concern. In much the way that some twenty-first-century educators are reluctant to teach children about birth control, fearing it might inadvertently encourage promiscuity, public health officials in the first half of the twentieth century were sometimes reluctant to educate people about how to avoid sexually transmitted diseases because then the illnesses would no longer serve as a deterrent to promiscuity (Brandt 1987, 46, 113; Parascandola 2008, 130). Abstinence, then, was the recommended preventative. Hemingway later lightly satirized his father's prudishness in "Fathers and Sons," the final story in the collection *Winner Take Nothing*, when young Nick Adams asks his father what "mashing" is: "His father had summed up the whole matter by stating that masturbation produced blindness, insanity, and death, while a man who went with prostitutes would contract hideous venereal diseases and that the thing to do was to keep your hands off of people" (1987, 371).
5. See Claude Caswell for a discussion of the significance of the prostitute in Hemingway's writings:

> The iconography of prostitution and the psychological idiosyncrasies of women working in the profession would also soon become a central trope in the young Hemingway's growing body of fiction. The prostitute "consciousness," as an ambivalent form of both social rebellion and "selling out"—establishment of a kind of courageous identity and yet at the same time a despairing loss of integrity—became in Hemingway's texts a key symbol of modernist reality (1998, 77–78).

6. If syphilis as a metaphor for evil seems overly melodramatic and Victorian for the modernist Hemingway, it's important to remember that decades later he wrote, in *A Moveable Feast*, "Some people show evil as a great race horse shows breeding. They have the dignity of a hard *chancre*" (*AMF* 109). A chancre is the sore that forms on the body near the point at which the infection entered the system (Hayden 2003, 53). For many patients, it is the first telltale symptom of syphilis.

7. Ironically, syphilis took the life of de Maupassant, whom Hemingway revered. The French writer was institutionalized after a suicide attempt and died when he was only 43 (Jobst and Williamson 1994, 53). See James J. Martine, Jack W. Jobst and W. J. Williamson, and Bryan Giemza (2010, especially 84–90) for discussions of de Maupassant's influence on Hemingway.
8. Interestingly, there was a historical precedent for this concept. Public health officials of the Progressive Era "appealed to enlightened capitalistic self-interest in their campaigns for extending public health facilities for venereal disease" (Brandt 1987, 134), citing the potential costs to employers: "The costs of venereally infected workers could often be hidden beyond the loss columns of the business ledger. Industrial accidents were often attributed to syphilis, with its dire impact on the neurological and cardiovascular systems. Public health officials frequently reminded businessmen of the costs of workmen's compensation for injuries incurred by syphilitics. Even more ominous, however, were the dangers of accidents not only to workers but to the public. A number of major train wrecks during the 1920s, for example, were attributed to advanced syphilis in the engineer." (134). Brandt notes, "Some corporations responded by creating anti-venereal programs for their workers" (134).
9. Edmund Wilson was the first to compare Hemingway to Goya, writing in 1924, "His bull-fight sketches have the dry sharpness and elegance of the bull-fight lithographs of Goya. And, like Goya, he is concerned first of all with making a fine picture" (1924, 223). See Emily Stipes Watts (1971, passim, but especially 57–65), Rudolf Haas, Jeffrey Meyers (1985, "Hemingway and Goya"), and Nancy R. Comley and Robert Scholes (1994, 114–18) for expanded discussions of the artistic relationships between Hemingway and Goya. Haas suggests that Hemingway's character El Sordo in the novel *For Whom the Bell Tolls* is an allusion to Goya, who owned a house named "Quinta del Sordo" (1987, 33). Haas contends that when El Sordo describes the hill on which he will die as "shaped like a chancre" (Hemingway 1940, 309), "Hemingway deliberately uses a clinical word" to express "the misery and hopelessness of the situation" and the "pessimistic attitude towards war and glory" that he and Goya shared (Haas 1987, 33).

References

Baker, Carlos. 1969. *Ernest Hemingway: A Life Story*. New York: Scribner's.

Birmingham, Kevin. 2014. *The Most Dangerous Book: The Battle for James Joyce's Ulysses*. New York: Penguin.

Bock, Martin. 1997. Syphilisation and Its Discontents: Somatic Indications of Psychological Ills in Joyce and Lowry. In *Joyce/Lowry: Critical Perspectives*, 126–144. Lexington: University Press of Kentucky.

Brand, Anthony. 2004. 'Far from Simple': The Published Photographs in *Death in the Afternoon*. In *A Companion to Hemingway's Death in the Afternoon*, ed. Miriam B. Mandel, 165–187. Rochester: Camden House.

Brandt, Allan M. 1987. *No Magic Bullet: A Social History of Venereal Disease in the United States Since 1880*. Expanded Edition. New York: Oxford University Press.

Brasch, James D., and Joseph Sigman. 1981. *Hemingway's Library: A Composite Record*. New York: Garland. John F. Kennedy Presidential Library and Museum.

Brian, Denis. 1988. *The True Gen: An Intimate Portrait of Hemingway—By Those Who Knew Him*. New York: Grove.

Burwell, Rose Marie. 1996. *Hemingway: The Postwar Years and the Posthumous Novels*. New York: Cambridge University Press.

Caswell, Claude. 1998. City of Brothelly Love: The Influence of Paris and Prostitution on Hemingway's Fiction. In *French Connections: Hemingway and Fitzgerald Abroad*, ed. J. Gerald Kennedy and Jackson R. Bryer, 75–100. New York: St. Martin's Press.

Cawthorne, Terence. 1962. Goya's Illness. *Proceedings of the Royal Society of Medicine* 55 (March): 213–217.

Comley, Nancy R., and Robert Scholes. 1994. *Hemingway's Genders: Rereading the Hemingway Text*. New Haven: Yale State University Press.

Donaldson, Scott. 1977. *By Force of Will: The Life and Art of Ernest Hemingway*. New York: Viking.

Eide, Marian. 1998. Beyond 'Syphilisation': *Finnegans Wake*, AIDS, and the Discourse of Contagion. In *Quare Joyce*, ed. Joseph Valente, 225–240. Ann Arbor: University of Michigan Press.

Felisati, D., and G. Sperati. 2010. Francisco Goya and His Illness. *Acta Otorhinolaryngologica Italica* 30: 264–270.

Ferris, Kathleen. 1995. *James Joyce and the Burden of Disease*. Lexington: University Press of Kentucky.

Fuentes, Norberto. 1984. *Hemingway in Cuba*. Secaucus: Lyle Stuart, Inc.

Giemza, Bryan. 2010. The French Connection: Some Visual and Literary Sources for the French Connection in Hemingway's 'The Light of the World. *Hemingway Review* 30 (1 Fall): 84–102.

Goya, Francisco. 2015. Plate 15 from 'Disasters of War' (*Los Desastres de la Guerra*: And there is no help (*Y no hai remedio*). In *The Collection Online*. Metropolitan Museum of Art.

Haas, Rudolf. 1987. Hemingway and Goya: 'Boundary Situations' and their Representation in Literature and the Arts. *Yearbook of Comparative and General Literature* 36: 29–40.

Hayden, Deborah. 2003. *Pox: Genius, Madness, and the Mysteries of Syphilis*. New York: Basic Books.

Hays, Peter L. 1995. Hemingway's Clinical Depression: A Speculation. *Hemingway Review* 14 (2): 50–63.

Hemingway, Ernest. 1925. *In Our Time*. New York: Collier.

———. 1926. *The Sun Also Rises*. New York: Collier.

———. 1929. *A Farewell to Arms*. New York: Simon & Schuster.

———. 1932. *Death in the Afternoon*. New York: Scribner's.

———. 1934. Introduction to *Quintanilla*. New York: Pierre Matisse Gallery. Reprinted in *Hemingway and the Mechanism of Fame*, edited by Matthew J. Bruccoli. Columbia, South Carolina: University of South Carolina Press, 31–34.

———. 1937. *To Have and Have Not*. New York: Scribner's.

———. 1940. *For Whom the Bell Tolls*. New York: Collier.

———. 1950. *Across the River and into the Trees*. New York: Scribners.

———. (1970) 1972. *Islands in the Stream*. New York: Bantam.

———. 1981. *Ernest Hemingway: Selected Letters, 1917–1961*, ed. Carlos Baker. New York: Scribner's.

———. 1987. *The Complete Short Stories of Ernest Hemingway: The Finca Vigia Edition*. New York: Scribner.

———. 2005. *Under Kilimanjaro*, ed. Robert W. Lewis and Robert E. Fleming. Kent: Kent State University Press.

Iuliano, Fiorenzo. 2014. Staging the Stigma: Syphilis and Its Metaphors in Claude McKay's *The Clinic*. *StatusQuaestionis: A Journal of European and American Studies* 6: 40–62. http://www.jmes.uniroma1.it/index.php/statusquaestionis/article/download/12472/12467

Jobst, Jack W., and W.J. Williamson. 1994. Hemingway and Maupassant: More Light on 'The Light of the World.'. *Hemingway Review* 13 (2 Spring): 52–61.

Joyce, James. (1922) 1997. *Ulysses*. New York: Knopf.
Kadlec, David. 2000. *Mosaic Modernism: Anarchism, Pragmatism, Culture*. Baltimore: Johns Hopkins University Press.
Lyons, J.B. 1988. *Thrust Syphilis Down to Hell and Other Rejoyceana: Studies in the Border-Lands of Literature and Medicine*. Dublin: Glendale.
Mandel, Miriam B. 2004. Subject and Author: The Literary Backgrounds of *Death in the Afternoon*. In *A Companion to Hemingway's Death in the Afternoon*, ed. Miriam B. Mandel, 79–119. Rochester: Camden House.
Martine, James J. 1970. A Little Light on Hemingway's 'The Light of the World.'. *Studies in Short Fiction* 7: 465–467.
Meyers, Jeffrey. 1985. *Hemingway*. New York: Harper & Row.
Moddelmog, Debra A. 2013. Sex, Sexuality, and Marriage. In *Ernest Hemingway in Context*, ed. Debra Moddelmog and Suzanne del Gizzo, 357–366. Cambridge: New York.
Nickel, Matthew. 2013. Religion. In *Ernest Hemingway in Context*, ed. Debra Moddelmog and Suzanne del Gizzo, 347–356. Cambridge: New York.
Parascandola, John. 2008. *Sex, Sin, and Science: A History of Syphilis in America*. Westport: Praeger.
Porter, Laurence M. 1980. Syphilis as Muse in Thomas Mann's *Doctor Faustus*. In *Medicine and Literature*, ed. Enid Rhodes Peschel, 147–152. New York: Seale Watson.
Ravin, James G., and Tracy B. Ravin. 1999. What Ailed Goya? *Survey of Ophthalmology* 44 (September–October): 163–170.
Reynolds, Michael. [1981] 1996. *Hemingway's Reading, 1910–1940: An Inventory*. Princeton: Princeton University Press. John F. Kennedy Presidential Library and Museum.
———. 1996. *A Farewell to Arms*: Doctors in the House of Love. In *The Cambridge Companion to Ernest Hemingway*, ed. Scott Donaldson, 109–127. New York: Cambridge University Press.
Rütten, Thomas. 2013. Genius and Degenerate? Thomas Mann's *Doktor Faustus* and a Medical Discourse on Syphilis. In *Contagionism and Contagious Diseases: Medicine and Literature 1880–1933*, ed. Thomas Rütten and Martina King, 147–166. Berlin: De Gruyter.
Sanford, Marcelline Hemingway. 1999. *At the Hemingways, with Fifty Years of Correspondence between Ernest and Marcelline Hemingway*. Moscow: University of Idaho Press.

Smith, Paul. 1989. *A Reader's Guide to the Short Stories of Ernest Hemingway*. Boston: Hall.

Spilka, Mark. 1990. *Hemingway's Quarrel with Androgyny*. Lincoln: University of Nebraska Press.

Strychacz, Thomas F. 2004. *Hemingway's Theaters of Masculinity*. Baton Rouge: Louisiana State University Press.

Sweeney, Gerard M. 1998. Wharton's *Bewitched*. *Explicator* 56: 198–201.

Takano, Yasushi. n.d. *Against the Victorian Normalization of Sexuality: A Study of Hemingway's Representation of Syphilis*. Kyushu University. http://www2.lit.kyushuu.ac.jp/$takano/literature/syphilis.pdf

Timins, Michael. 2012. 'The Sisters': Their Disease. *James Joyce Quarterly* 49: 441–454.

Tyler, Lisa. 2016. 'Our Fathers Lied': The Great War and Paternal Betrayal in Hemingway's *In Our Time*. In *Teaching Hemingway and War*, ed. Alex Vernon, 30–40. Kent: Kent State University Press.

Waisbren, Burton A., and Florence L. Walzl. 1974. Paresis and the Priest: James Joyce's Symbolic Use of Syphilis in 'The Sisters.'. *Annals of Internal Medicine* 1974: 758–762.

Watts, Emily Stipes. 1971. *Ernest Hemingway and the Arts*. Urbana: University of Illinois Press.

Wilson, Edmund. 1924. Mr. Hemingway's Dry-Points. *The Dial* LXXVII.4 (October): 340–41. Reprinted in *Ernest Hemingway: Five Decades of Criticism*, edited by Linda Welshimer Wagner, 222–223. East Lansing: Michigan State University Press.

Index[1]

[1]Note: Page number followed by 'n' denotes to note.

K. Nixon, L. Servitje (eds.), *Syphilis and Subjectivity*,
https://doi.org/10.1007/978-3-319-66367-8

The manufacturer's authorised representative in the EU is Springer Nature Customer Service Centre GmbH, Europaplatz 3, 69115 Heidelberg, Germany. If you have any concerns regarding our products, please contact ProductSafety@springernature.com

Printed and bound by CPI Group (UK) Ltd, Croydon, CR0 4YY

30/09/2026

02225656-0002